RENAL DIET

RECIPES

The Comprehensive Cookbook for Renal Diet and How It Cures Kidney

(Medicinal Recipes for Healthy Kidney)

Martin Salas

Published by Alex Howard

© **Martin Salas**

All Rights Reserved

Renal Diet Recipes: The Comprehensive Cookbook for Renal Diet and How It Cures Kidney (Medicinal Recipes for Healthy Kidney)

ISBN 978-1-989891-87-2

Legal & Disclaimer

The information contained in this book is not designed to replace or take the place of any form of medicine or professional medical advice. The information in this book has been provided for educational and entertainment purposes only.

TABLE OF CONTENTS

Part 1

Introduction

When it comes to your health and well being, it's a good idea to see your doctor as often as possible to make sure you don't run into preventable problems that you needn't catch. The kidneys are your body's toxin filter (as is the liver), cleaning the blood of foreign substances and toxins that are released from things like preservatives in food and other toxins.

When you eat irresponsibly and fill your body with toxins, either from food, drinks (alcohol for example) or even from the air you breathe (free radicals are in the sun and transfer through your skin, through dirty air, and many foods contain them). Your body also tends to convert many things that seem benign until your body's organs convert them into things like formaldehyde due to a chemical reaction and morphing phase.

One example of this is most of those diet sugars used in diet sodas for example, Aspartame turns into Formaldehyde in the body. These toxins have to be removed or they can lead to disease, renal (kidney) failure, cancer, and various other painful problems.

What is renal or kidney failure? This is when your kidneys are not capable of ridding the body of the toxins and wastes in your blood from the foods you eat and the things you drink. This is also called "chronic kidney disease" or "chronic renal failure".

This is not a condition that happens overnight- it is a progressive problem and in that it can be both discovered early and treated, diet changed, and resolving what is causing the problem is possible. It's possible to have partial renal failure but usually it takes a lot of time (or really bad diet for a short time) to reach total renal failure. You don't want to reach total renal failure because this will require regular dialysis treatments to save your life.

Dialysis treatments specifically clean the blood of waste and toxins in the blood using a machine because your body can no longer do the job. Without treatments you could die a very painful death. Renal failure can be the result of long term diabetes, high blood pressure, irresponsible diet, and can stem out of other health concerns.

A renal diet is about moderating the intake of protein and phosphorus in your diet. Limiting your sodium intake is also important. By controlling these two factors you can control most of the toxins/waste created by your body and in turn this helps your kidney function. If you catch this early enough and really moderate your diet with extreme care, you could prevent total renal failure. If you catch this early you can eliminate the problem completely.

What Is A Renal Diet?

A Renal diet is an eating plan worked out to help people suffering from renal diseases to boost the effectiveness of treatment by minimizing the levels of waste products in their blood.

The renal diet is designed to cause as little extra work or stress on the damaged kidneys as possible, while still providing sufficient good nutrients and energy that the body needs.

A renal diet follows several basic guidelines. The first guideline is that it must be a balanced, healthy and sustainable diet, rich in fibers, vitamins, natural grains, carbohydrates, omega 3 fats and fluids. Proteins should be adequate, but not excessive.

The salts that are likely to accumulate in the bloodstream, are kept to a minimum. Blood electrolyte levels are monitored regularly and the diet adjusted accordingly. It is very important to follow specific advice from your doctor and dietitian.

Renal diet guidelines are built around blood test results and a normal healthy balanced diet. The idea is to limit the intake of salts that are too high. Fluids may also be restricted if your kidneys are unable to excrete sufficient water. Protein intake is limited so wastes like urea are kept at a minimum.

The salts that commonly need to be restricted are:

Sodium. Sodium can cause high blood pressure and fluid retention. Most renal diets use minimal salt in cooking, and stipulate, "No added salts". "Lo-salt" combinations are not suitable for salt replacement as they have high potassium levels, and should not be used. Processed foods, sausages, sauces, ketchup's and many canned foods should be avoided.

Phosphorus cannot be removed by dialysis, so it might become a problem. Levels are monitored, and kept under control by diet and sometimes medication. High phosphorus foods include dairy products, beans, peas, beer and cola drinks.

Potassium should only be restricted if the blood levels are high. Many healthy vegetables and fruits contain potassium. High potassium foods include apricots, orange juice, bananas, avocados, beets, spinach and many more.

Proteins are a necessary part of a healthy diet, but should only be eaten in small amounts. Proteins that should be restricted, include all meats, fish, eggs and dairy products.

Fluids might be restricted if water retention is present in the form of generalized swelling or fluid in the lungs. Fluids are often strictly controlled for patients on haemodialysis. Fluids include all beverages, soups, water and juices.

Carbohydrates are energy foods and should not be restricted unless you are a diabetic or overweight. Lastly, it might be advisable to take vitamin and antioxidant supplements to boost your immune system.

Benefits Of A Healthy Renal Diet To Kidney

It is the role of your kidneys to filter out things you don't need and to maintain a balance of the good things your body needs. If your kidneys can't play this role efficiently what can you do to get toxic substances from your body? A Doctor recommended renal diet could help you filter out toxic substances you don't need in your body.

A healthy renal diet means less taxation of your kidneys
Apart from eliminating urine and other toxic substances such as ammonia, your kidneys help the body to create red blood cells and to keep blood pressure steady. A Doctor recommended diet ensures your kidneys have a lesser workload to handle. This happens through the control of toxic substances intake. Some of the leading substances that add toxins in your blood stream and cause problems for your kidneys are; sodium, potassium, some proteins, and phosphorous. A Doctor monitored dietary regime will ensure that these substances are eliminated completely from your diet or they are taken in moderation.

A renal diet helps you to prevent the progression of renal failure.
You want to make sure that your kidney problem does not develop into kidney failure. A healthy diet as recommended by your doctor plays a major role in the management of your kidney disease such that it doesn't grow out of control.

A healthy renal diet can indeed help you to manage this problem.
The aim of the Doctor is to help you filter toxic substances long before they get in your body. Toxic substances get into your body through the food you eat. If you can avoid eating foods that contain toxic substances you will be able lessen the burden on your kidneys to flash out unwanted things from your blood stream. The benefit of following a healthy diet is feeling good and having more energy

A Renal Diet Helps in the Control of Phosphorous and Potassium Levels in your Body

A healthy diet helps you to limit protein to the right amount, and to maintain bone strength by making sure there isn't too much phosphorous in your bloodstream. It also ensures that there is no excess potassium in your system because it can adversely affect your heartbeat.

A renal diet ensures that the level of sodium in your body is under strict control in order to avoid water retention. If fluids are retained in your body as a result of excessive sodium intake, you shall suffer a lot of pain due to swellings around leg joints.

The Do's and Don'ts of a Kidney Diet

If you are suffering from a renal problem such as kidney stones, then you may be interested to know that a kidney diet plays a significant part in mitigating adverse symptoms and helping the kidney recover quickly from the problem. While some foods may be very nutritious and good for the body, they may pose serious problems to the kidneys in the long run. Therefore, it is well-advised to eat meals in moderation and also evaluating the suitability of the diet to your condition.

A kidney diet should avoid calcium and phosphorous enriched foods

At best, dietary changes such as avoidance of calcium and phosphorous rich foods will become necessary if certain kidney problems are at a critical stage. This applies mostly to individuals who are at risk of developing a renal disorder.

Below are some of the do's and don'ts that you should consider when planning your kidney diet.

Don'ts of a kidney diet

- Don't use food recipes in your diet for renal disease which have substantial quantities of mineral salts especially oxalate salts from calcium, phosphorus, manganese. These mineral elements can cause faster kidney degeneration and severe impairment to kidney functioning.
- Don't eat excess portions of foods which have high concentrations of saturated fats such as fries, burgers, and red meat or any processed foods.
- Don't drink alcohol, energy drinks, or beverages with high sugar content-both may overwork the liver and worsen or cause degeneration of the kidney problem.
- Don't consume sugary substances such as, snacks, deserts, or candies because they cause dehydration and overwork the kidney just like salts.
- Do not take all kinds of natural red meat in your kidney diet-beef, pork, bacon, or mutton and their alternatives fried, cured, or processed meats, instead look for lean white meat from poultry.
- Do not use any artificial sweeteners when preparing foods because they have no nutritional benefits
- Do not use margarine or mayonnaise but alternatives such as avocado fruit if you want to consume fat.

- Do not eat more helpings than necessary especially in regard to delicacies such as fries, ice creams, sodas, and other sweet foods an all kinds of processed or canned foods
- Don't consume more carbohydrates than necessary in your kidney diet and this includes such carbs like pasta, white rice, biscuits, white sugar, white rice, and pasta.

Do's of a kidney diet

- Do take enough fluids to keep concentration of minerals such as calcium and sodium on the kidney low. These will to ensure proper kidney functioning, prevent dehydration which is the common cause of kidney stones in the renal tubes, and detoxify the kidney as well.

- Do adopt a balanced diet for renal disease which comprises fresh vegetables, whole grains, and lean meat as well as water. Greens and fruits rich in vitamins improve cell metabolism and functioning of organs.

- Do take fiber or incorporate fibre rich meals and whole grains in your renal diet which are low in carbs but promote general health and boost kidney functioning.

- Do eat moderately and develop healthy eating habits to ensure that your body gets the right supply of minerals and nutrients.

- Do eat vegetables and fruits as often as you can and incorporate them in your kidney diet plan to boost your immunity and cell metabolism

- Do use low-fat milk products such as milk powder if you have to use them instead of using milk with cream or fat.

- Do use mono unsaturated fat or natural fat when cooking and lower the amount of fat that you consume per day in your meals.

- Do embrace active and vibrant life to reduce obesity or abnormal weight, boost functioning of renal diet, and promote good body metabolism and kidney functioning. Exercise ensures blood circulation to kidney and boosts activities such as detoxification and filtering.

Renal diet recipes

1 Slow-Cooked Lemon Chicken

Light and lemony, this slow-cooker chicken recipe re?uires little prep and minimal ingredients to make moist, tender chicken breasts. A perfect slow-cooker meal anytime, it's especially nice for spring and summer.

Serves 4 (1 serving = 4 ounces)

Ingredients

- 1 teaspoon dried oregano
- ¼ teaspoon ground black pepper
- 2 tablespoons butter, unsalted
- 1 pound chicken breast, boneless, skinless
- ¼ cup chicken broth, low sodium
- ¼ cup water
- 1 tablespoon lemon juice
- 2 cloves garlic, minced
- 1 teaspoon fresh basil, chopped

Instructions

- Combine oregano and ground black pepper in a small bowl. Rub mixture on the chicken.
- Melt the butter in a medium-sized skillet over medium heat. Brown the chicken in the melted butter and then transfer the chicken to the slow cooker.

- Place chicken broth, water, lemon juice and garlic in the skillet. Bring it to a boil so it loosens the browned bits from the skillet. Pour over the chicken.
- Cover, set slow cooker on high for 2½ hours or low for 5 hours.
- Add basil and baste chicken. Cover, cook on high for an additional 15–30 minutes or until chicken is tender

Nutrition Info

Calories 197 cal
Total Fat 9 g
Saturated Fat 5 g
Trans Fat 0 g

2 Zesty Orange Tilapia

Fresh orange zest gives this mild and succulent fish a citrusy flavor boost. Julienned veggies add texture for a simple and delicious meal.

Serves 4 (1 serving = 4 ounces)

Ingredients

- 16 ounces tilapia
- 1 cup carrots, julienned
- ¾ cup celery, julienned
- ½ cup green onions, sliced
- 2 teaspoons grated orange peel (zest)
- 4 teaspoons orange juice
- 1 teaspoon ground black pepper

Instructions

- Preheat oven to 450° F.
- In a small bowl, mix carrots, celery, green onions and orange zest together.
- Cut the tilapia into 4 equal portions. Tear off 4 large squares of foil and spray foil with nonstick spray.
- Place ¼ of the vegetables on each piece of the foil slightly off center and top with the fish. Sprinkle 1 teaspoon of orange juice on top of each. Season with ground black pepper.
- Fold the foil over and crimp the edges to make an envelope or pouch and place the foil packets on a baking sheet. Bake for about 12 minutes (3–5 minutes longer if the fish is thick). Fish should separate easily with a fork when done.
- Remove the pouches and place directly onto the plates. Be careful when opening due to the steam.

Nutrition Info

Calories 133 cal
Total Fat 2 g
Carbohydrates 6 g
Protein 24 g
Phosphorus 214 mg
Potassium 543 mg
Dietary Fiber 1.7 g
Calcium 42 mg

3 Herb-Crusted Roast Leg of Lamb

Prep/Cook Time:
Serves: 12 (1 serving = 4 ounces)

Ingredients

- 1 4-pound leg of lamb
- 3 tablespoons lemon juice
- 1 tablespoon curry powder
- 2 cloves garlic, minced
- ½ teaspoon ground black pepper
- 1 cup onions, sliced
- ½ cup dry vermouth

Instructions

- Preheat oven to 400° F.
- Place leg of lamb on a roasting pan. Sprinkle with 1 teaspoon of lemon juice.
- Make paste with 2 teaspoons of lemon juice and the rest of the spices. Rub the paste onto the lamb.
- Roast lamb in 400° F oven for 30 minutes.
- Drain off fat and add vermouth and onions.
- Reduce heat to 325° F and cook for an additional 1¾–2 hours. Baste leg of lamb frequently. When internal temperature is 145° F, remove from oven and let rest 3 minutes before serving.

Nutrition Info

Calories 292 cal
Total Fat 20 g
Phosphorus 232 mg
Potassium 419 mg
Dietary Fiber 0 g
Calcium 19 mg

4. 60-Second Salsa

Prep/Cook Time: 1 min
8 servings

Ingredients

- 4 roma or plum tomatoes, chopped
- 2 green onions, chopped
- 3 garlic cloves, minced
- 1/2 - 1 green bell pepper, chopped
- 1/2 - 1 fresh jalapeño, chopped
- 1/2 bunch fresh cilantro, chopped
- 1/2 teaspoon cumin
- 1/4 cup fresh oregano, chopped or 1 tablespoon dried

Instructions
- Mix all ingredients in a food processor or blender until the larger items are small and chunky.
- Let sit for a couple of hours in the refrigerator.
- Best served chilled and with plain tortilla chips.

Nutrition Info
Calories 14
Carbohydrates 2 g
Protein 1 g
Dietary Fiber 0 g
Fat 1 g

5. 40-Second Omelet

Prep/Cook Time: 30 mins
Serves: 1

Ingredients

- 2 eggs
- 2 tablespoons water
- 1 tablespoon unsalted butter
- 1/2 cup filling (vegetable, meat, seafood)

Instructions

- Beat together eggs and water until blended.
- In a 10-inch omelet pan or fry pan, heat butter until just hot enough to sizzle a drop of water.
- Pour in egg mixture. Mixture should set at edges right away. With an inverted pancake turner, carefully push cooked portions at edges toward center so uncooked portions can reach the hot pan surface. Tilt pan and move as necessary.
- Continue until egg is set and will not flow. Fill the omelet with 1/2 cup of vegetable, meat, seafood, or fruit filling, if desired. Put filling on left side if you're right handed and the right side if you're left handed.
- With the pancake turner, fold omelet in half. Invert onto a plate with the omelet's bottom side facing up.

Nutrition Info

Calories 255
Carbohydrates 1.3 g
Protein 13 g
Dietary Fiber 2 g
Sodium 145 mg

6 Hawaiian-Style Slow-Cooked Pulled Pork

Prep/Cook Time: 5 hrs

Serves 16

Ingredients

- 4 pounds pork roast
- ½ teaspoon ground black pepper
- ½ teaspoon paprika
- 1 teaspoon onion powder
- ½ teaspoon garlic powder
- 2 tablespoons liquid smoke
- Optional garnish: (pickled red onions or radishes) 1 red onion or 4 radishes, ⅓ cup white vinegar and ¼ teaspoon of sugar

Instructions

- Combine black pepper, paprika, onion and garlic powder in a small bowl.
- Rub the seasoning blend on all sides of the pork. Place pork into a slow cooker or a crock-pot. Sprinkle with liquid smoke.
- Add enough water to the slow cooker or crock-pot to measure ¼–½" deep. Cook on high for 4–5 hours.
- Remove pork from cooking liquid and shred meat using two forks.
- Optional: Garnish with sliced pickled red onions or radishes.

Tip: For quick pickled red onions or radishes, marinate one sliced red onion or 4 sliced radishes in a ⅓ cup of white vinegar and a ¼ teaspoon of sugar for 1 hour. Drain and use as a garnish.

Nutrition Info

Calories 285 cal
Total Fat 21 g
Saturated Fat 7 g
Trans Fat 0 g

Cholesterol 83 mg
Sodium 54 mg
Carbohydrates 1 g
Protein 20 g

7 Roast Pork Loin With Sweet and Tart Apple Stuffing

Prep/Cook Time: 1 hr, 15 min
Serves 6

Ingredients
- Cherry Marmalade Glaze:
- ½ cup sugar-free orange marmalade
- ¼ cup apple juice
- ¼ cup dried cherries
- 1/8 teaspoon cinnamon
- 1/8 teaspoon nutmeg
- Apple Stuffing:
- 2 tablespoons canola oil
- 2 cups packed cubed Hawaiian rolls (or any white bread)
- ½ cup finely diced Granny Smith, Macintosh or Honey Crisp apple
- 2 tablespoons unsalted butter
- 2 tablespoons finely diced onions
- 2 tablespoons finely diced celery
- 1 tablespoon fresh thyme or ½ teaspoon dried thyme
- 1 teaspoon black pepper
- ½ cup low-sodium chicken stock

Roast Pork Loin:

- 1 pound Hormel® natural boneless pork loin
- 2 18-inch pieces of butcher twine

Instructions

Cherry Marmalade Glaze:

- Mix all glaze ingredients in a small saucepan on medium-high heat until marmalade is melted and starts to simmer. Turn off heat and set aside.
- Preheat oven to 400° F.
- Sauté all ingredients in canola oil except for chicken stock for 2–3 minutes in large sauté pan on medium-high heat.
- Slowly add chicken stock until moist, but not too wet. (You may not need it all, depending on how much juice is released from the apples during cooking.)
- Remove from heat and chill to room temperature.
- Meanwhile, cut five slits about 1 inch apart along the length of the loin, forming several pockets.
- Stuff each pocket with about 2 tablespoons of stuffing (there should be a little left over).
- Tie one long piece of twine around the length of the loin and tie additional twine across the shorter length as needed to keep the stuffing in place.
- Place remaining stuffing on a baking sheet tray, place tied stuffed pork on top and bake for 45 minutes at 400° F or until you reach an internal temperature of 160° F.
- Spoon on the dried cherry marmalade glaze, shut oven heat off and let rest in oven for 10–15 minutes. Remove pork loin, slice into portions then serve.

Nutrition Info

Calories 263 cal
Total Fat 14 g
Saturated Fat 4 g
Trans Fat 0 g
Cholesterol 50 mg
Sodium 137 mg
Carbohydrates 22 g
Protein 14 g

8 Low Potassium Potatoes

Prep/Cook Time: 20 minutes
Serving: 4

Ingredients

Method One:
- potatoes - peeled and cut into slices
Method Two:
- potatoes - peeled and diced into 1cm cubes

Instructions

Method One:

- 'Double boiled' potatoes
- Peel the potatoes and cut into thin slices
- Bring to the boil, using four times as much water as potatoes
- Throw water away, and replace with the same volume of fresh boiling water
- When cooked, drain and measure your allowance

Method Two:

- Peel and dice potatoes into 1cm cubes
- Bring to boil in 10 times as much water as potatoes
- Cook until potatoes are soft

Nutrition Info

Calories 189 cal
Total Fat 11 g
Saturated Fat 3 g
Trans Fat 0.5 g
Cholesterol 30 mg
Sodium 125 mg
Carbohydrates 12 g
Protein 11 g

9 Chicken Curry

Prep/Cook Time: 1 hr 20 minutes
Serving: 4

Ingredients

- chicken - 450g (18oz)
- garlic, crushed - 1 small clove
- onion - 1 medium (150g / 6oz)

- vegetable oil - 1 tablespoon
- water - Approx ½ pint (284ml)
- black pepper - ¼ teaspoon
- curry powder - 1 tablespoon
- flour - 1 dessertspoon
- margarine - 1oz (25g)

Instructions

- Dice the chicken.
- Fry the onion and garlic until brown in vegetable oil.
- Add the chicken and fry gently.
- In a separate pan, melt the margarine and whisk in the flour to make a roux. Add a little water while doing this to form a paste.
- Add in remaining water, and whisk in curry powder & pepper. Add sauce to chicken mix and allow come to the boil.
- Reduce heat, cover and simmer to allow sauce to thicken (20 minutes). Add more water if required to prevent burning.

Nutrition Info

Calories 190 cal
Total Fat 13 g
Saturated Fat 3 g
Trans Fat 0.7 g
Cholesterol 30 mg
Sodium 125 mg
Carbohydrates 12 g
Protein 21 g

10 Sauce-less BBQ Baby Back Ribs

Prep/Cook Time: 2 hrs, 45 min
Serves 12

Ingredients

- 2 slabs (about 3½ pounds) baby back ribs
- 12 mini-ears corn on the cob, fresh or frozen
- 1 portion of rub
- Chef McCargo's BBQ Spice Rub (mix all ingredients together):
- 1 cup packed dark brown sugar
- 1 teaspoon black pepper
- 1 teaspoon red pepper flakes
- 1 teaspoon smoked paprika
- 2 teaspoons granulated garlic = substitution Garlic Powder
- 2 teaspoons dehydrated onion flakes
- 2 teaspoons dark chili powder

Instructions

- Preheat oven to 400° F.

- Rub down both slabs of ribs on both sides with rub mixture.
- Place ribs on wire rack-lined tray. Wrap tightly with aluminum foil and bake for 1½ to 2 hours.
- Remove from oven and take off foil. Using tongs, set ribs aside. Drain liquids from the pan, then place ribs back on tray.
- Cook for an additional 15 minutes or until desired crispness.
- Let rest for 5–10 minutes, then cut and serve.

- To microwave corn on the cob, use a microwave-safe 9" x 9" casserole pan. Stand all the mini-ears of corn on end in the dish. Pour about ½ inch of water into the dish. Cover tightly with plastic wrap. Microwave 5–7 minutes on high.

TIP:

* Make extra spice rub and use it to kick up the flavor of beef or chicken.

* Cook ribs at 250° F (curled side of ribs facing up) for the first 3 hours, then increase the temperature to 300° F for the final 3 hours.
* To grill corn on the cob, shuck each ear of corn, removing husk and any remaining silk strands. Wrap the corn in aluminum foil and place on the grill for approximately 25 minutes, turning occasionally, until corn is tender.

Nutrition Info

Calories 324 cal
Total Fat 15 g
Saturated Fat 5 g
Trans Fat 0 g
Cholesterol 58 mg
Sodium 102 mg
Carbohydrates 33 g
Protein 18 g

11 Acorn Squash Baked with Pineapple

Prep/Cook Time: 1 hr
Serves: 2

Ingredients

- 1 acorn squash, cut in half and seeded
- 2 teaspoons + 1 tablespoon unsalted butter
- 2 teaspoons brown sugar
- 3 tablespoons pineapple, crushed
- 1/4 teaspoon nutmeg

Instructions

- Preheat oven to 400 degrees.
- Place squash with cut side up in greased baking pan.
- Place one teaspoon butter plus one teaspoon brown sugar in each acorn half.
- Cover squash with aluminum foil and bake until tender, approximately 30 minutes.
- Scoop cooked squash out of shells, leaving 1/4 inch thick shell.
- Mix cooked squash, pineapple, 1 tablespoon butter, and nutmeg. Beat until smooth.
- Spoon mixture into shells; heat at 425 degrees for approximately 15 minutes.

Nutrition Info

Calories 202
Carbohydrates 31 g
Protein 2 g
Sodium 90 mg
Potassium 783 mg
Phosphorus 80 mg

12 Alaska Baked Macaroni and Cheese

Prep/Cook Time: 30 min
Serves: 8

Ingredients

- 3 cups elbow, small shell or bowtie pasta
- 2 tablespoons flour
- 2 tablespoons unsalted butter
- 2 cups milk
- 1 teaspoon mustard powder
- 1 teaspoon paprika
- 1 tablespoon fresh thyme or tarragon, chopped or 1 teaspoon dry
- 2 cups cheese (gouda, cheddar, or any combo)
- croutons or chopped almonds to taste

Instructions

- Heat oven to 350 degrees.
- Boil pasta in a large pot until al-dente.
- Meanwhile, in a medium glass measuring cup, measure flour and butter. Microwave about 1-2 minutes until golden brown.
- Slowly stir in milk and continue microwaving until thickened. Stir in spices and herbs.
- Mix drained noodles, sauce, and cheese and put in a greased casserole dish. Bake about 20 minutes.
- Top with croutons or chopped almonds in the last 5 minutes.

Nutrition Info

Calories 424
Carbohydrates 36 g
Protein 22 g
Dietary Fiber 2g
Fat 20g
Sodium 479 mg
Potassium 237 mg
Phosphorus 428 mg

13 Alfredo Sauce

Serves: 8

Ingredients

- 1/4 cup olive oil
- 3 tablespoons all-purpose flour
- 1 clove garlic, minced
- 2 cups rice milk
- 4 ounces cream cheese
- 1/3 cup shredded Parmesan cheese
- 1/4 teaspoon ground nutmeg
- 1 tablespoon lemon juice

Instructions

- Heat olive oil in a large skillet over medium heat. Add flour and whisk to make a paste then add minced garlic.
- Slowly add rice milk, whisking constantly to prevent lumps. Let mixture come to a boil and thicken.

- Add cream cheese and mix well. Remove from heat.
- Add 1/3 cup Parmesan cheese, nutmeg, and lemon juice. Mix well.
- Serve over pasta, chicken, steamed vegetables, etc.

Nutrition Info

Calories 173
Carbohydrates 9 g
Protein 3 g
Sodium 142 mg
Potassium 32 mg
Phosphorus 75 mg

14 Almond Pecan Caramel Corn

Serves: 10

Ingredients

- 20 cups popped popcorn or about 3/4 cup popcorn kernels
- 2 cups unblanched almonds
- 1 cup pecan halves
- 1 cup granulated sugar
- 1 cup unsalted butter
- 1/2 cup corn syrup
- pinch of cream of tartar
- 1 teaspoon baking soda

Instructions

- In a large roasting pan, layer cooked popcorn evenly with almonds and pecans.
- In large heavy saucepan, stir together sugar, butter, corn syrup and cream of tartar.
- Bring to boil over medium-high heat, stirring constantly. Let boil for 5 minutes without stirring.
- Remove from heat and stir in baking soda.
- Pour caramel evenly over popcorn mixture, stirring to coat well.
- Bake at 200 degrees for 1 hour, stirring every 10 minutes.
- Let cool, stirring occasionally. Store in airtight tin for up to one week.

Nutrition Info

Calories 604
Carbohydrates 51 g
Protein 8 g
Dietary Fiber 4 g
Fat 6 g
Sodium 149 mg
Potassium 285 mg
Phosphorus 201 mg

15 Anytime Energy Bars

Prep/Cook Time: 50 mins
Serves: 8

Ingredients

- 1 cup rolled oats
- 1/2 teaspoon ground cinnamon
- 3 tablespoons unsalted peanuts, chopped
- 1/4 cup semi-sweet mini chocolate chips
- 1/3 cup shredded coconut
- 3 large eggs
- 1/3 cup applesauce
- 3 tablespoons honey

Instructions

- Heat oven to 325 degrees. Grease a 9×9 inch pan with cooking spray.
- In a large mixing bowl, combine oats, cinnamon, peanuts, chocolate chips and coconut.
- Beat eggs in a small mixing bowl. Add applesauce and honey and mix well.
- Add egg mixture to the oat mixture and mix well.
- Press mixture evenly into bottom of the greased 9×9 pan.
- Cook for 40 minutes. Cool, and then cut into bars.
- May keep refrigerated in an airtight container for up to one week.

Nutrition Info

Calories 206
Carbohydrates 27 g
Protein 7 g
Dietary Fiber 8 g

16 Apple & Cherry Chutney

Prep/Cook Time: 25 mins
Serves: 32

Ingredients

- 1 medium tart apple
- 1 cup dried tart cherries
- 1 small red onion, thinly sliced
- 1 cup apple cider vinegar
- 1 1/2 cups sugar

Instructions

- Quarter and core the apple and cut into thin slices, leaving the skin on.
- Put the apples and cherries in a heavy saucepan with the onions, vinegar, and sugar. Cook, stirring until the sugar is dissolved and the mixture is beginning to boil.
- Cover and reduce heat to low and cook until the onions are tender and the dried cherries are plump and tender, about 8-10 minutes.
- Uncover and bring the heat up to high and boil until the syrup around the fruit is reduced to a shiny glaze, about 5 minutes more. Chutney may be served at once or kept, covered and refrigerated for several days.

Nutrition Info

Calories 55
Carbohydrates 14 g
Protein < 1 g

Sodium 2 mg

17 BBQ Rub For Pork or Chicken

Prep/Cook Time: 10 min
Serves: 4

Ingredients

- 1 tablespoon brown sugar
- 1 teaspoon smoked paprika
- 1 teaspoon chili powder
- 1 teaspoon garlic, granulated
- 1 teaspoon onion powder
- 1 teaspoon cumin
- 1/4 teaspoon dry mustard powder
- 1/8 teaspoon allspice
- 1/8 teaspoon ground red pepper (optional)

Instructions
- In a bowl, blend all ingredients together thoroughly.
- Rub on pork or chicken before cooking.

Nutrition Info

Calories 20
Carbohydrates 4 g
Protein 0 g
Dietary Fiber 0 g
Sodium 9 mg

18 Beef Barley Soup

Prep/Cook Time: 15 mins
Serves: 10

Ingredients

- 1/2 teaspoon black pepper
- 2 lbs beef stew meat, diced 1 inch cubes
- 1/4 cup vegetable oil, divided
- 1 cup chopped onion
- 1/2 cup sliced mushrooms
- 2 carrots, diced
- 1/2 teaspoon garlic, minced
- 1/4 teaspoon dried thyme
- 1 can (14.5 ounces) chicken broth, low sodium
- 3 cups water
- 1 frozen package (16 ounces) of vegetables
- 2 potatoes, soaked and diced
- 1/2 cup barley

Instructions

- Season beef with pepper.
- Add 2 tablespoons oil to stew pot and saute 5 minutes.
- Add 2 more tablespoons of oil and add onions, carrots and mushrooms.
- Saute for 5 minutes and stir often.
- Add garlic and thyme and saute for 3 mins.
- Add chicken broth and water to pot.
- Add mixed vegtables, potatoes and barley.

- Stir and bring to boil.
- Cover and reduce heat.
- Simmer 1 to 1 1/2 hours.

Nutrition Info

Calories 270
Carbohydrates 22 g
Protein 23 g
Dietary Fiber 10 g
Sodium 105 mg
Potassium 678 mg
Phosphorus 250 mg

19 Biscuits with Master Mix

Prep/Cook Time: 20 mins
Serves: 12

Ingredients

- 3 cups Master Mix
- 2/3 cup Water

Instructions
- Preheat oven to 450 degrees.
- Combine ingredients and blend well.
- Let stand 5 minutes.
- On lightly floured board, knead dough about 15 times.
- Roll out to 1/2 inch thickness and cut with flour cutter until you have 12 biscuits.
- Place 2 inches apart on ungreased baking sheet.

- Bake 10-12 minutes until golden brown.

Nutrition Info
Calories 174
Carbohydrates 18 g
Protein 3 g
Dietary Fiber 10 g
Sodium 171 mg
Potassium 81 mg
Phosphorus 51 mg

20 Buttermilk Herb Ranch Dressing

Prep/Cook Time: 10 mins
Serves: 2

Ingredients

- 1/2 cup mayonnaise
- 1/2 cup milk
- 2 tablespoons vinegar
- 1 tablespoon fresh chives, chopped
- 1 tablespoon dill
- 1 tablespoon oregano leaves, chopped
- 1/4 teaspoon garlic powder

Instructions

- In a medium bowl, whisk mayonnaise, milk and vinegar.
- Then add fresh chives, dill, and oregano leaves with 1/4 teaspoon garlic powder.

- Mix together.
- Chill at least one hour to allow flavors to develop.
- Stir dressing well before serving.

Nutrition Info

Calories 83
Carbohydrates 1 g
Protein 1 g
Sodium 64 mg
Potassium 9 mg
Phosphorus 1 mg

21 Chicken 'n Orange Salad Sandwich

Prep/Cook Time: 15 mins
Serves: 6

Ingredients

- 1 cup chopped cooked chicken
- 1/2 cup celery, diced
- 1/2 cup green pepper, chopped
- 1/4 cup onion, finely sliced
- 1 cup Mandarin oranges
- 1/3 cup mayonnaise

Instructions
- Toss chicken, celery, green pepper, and onion to mix.
- Add mandarin oranges and mayonnaise.
- Mix gently.
- Serve on bread.

Nutrition Info

Calories 170
Carbohydrates 6 g
Protein 12 g
Sodium 97 mg
Potassium 241 mg
Phosphorus 106 mg

22 Blasted Brussels Sprouts

Prep/Cook Time: 10 mins
Serves: 4-6

Ingredients

- 2 cups Brussels Sprouts (about one stalk)
- 1-2 tablespoons olive oil
- 2-4 tablespoons fresh grated Parmesan Cheese
- 1/4 cup fruit or herb flavored vinegar

Instructions

- Preheat oven to 450 degrees.
- Clean off old leaves. Cut larger sprouts in half and leave smaller sprouts whole.
- Toss sprouts with olive oil.
- Put on lightly oiled baking sheet.
- Roast about 10 minutes. Sprouts are done when tender to pierce with a fork.
- Remove from oven, sprinkle with fruit vinegar and freshly grated Parmesean cheese

Nutrition Info

Calories 68
Carbohydrates 4 g
Protein 3 g
Dietary Fiber 5 g
Sodium 70 mg
Potassium 182 mg
Phosphorus 59 mg

23 Caramel Custard

Prep/Cook Time: 1 hr 20 mins
Serves: 6

Ingredients

- 2 tablespoons sugar
- 2 tablespoons water
- 6 eggs
- 4 drops vanilla extract
- 1/2 cup + 2 tablespoons sugar
- 3 cups 2% milk

Instructions

- To make the caramel, place sugar and water in heat-proof dish and place in a microwave.
- Cook for 4 minutes on high or until the sugar is caramelized.
- To make on the stove, melt sugar and water in pan until pale gold in color.

- Pour into a 5 cup souffle or baking dish.
- Let cool.
- Preheat oven to 350 degrees.
- To make the custard, break eggs into medium mixing bowl; whisk until frothy.
- Stir in vanilla extract.
- Gradually add sugar and then milk, whisking continuously.
- Pour custard over the top of the caramel.
- Cook in preheated oven 35-40 minutes.
- Remove from oven and let cool about 30 minutes or until set.
- Loosen custard from sides of the dish with a knife. Place serving dish upside-down on top of souffle dish and invert, giving a gentle shake.
- Arrange choice of fruit around caramel and serve. Choices include orange rings and banana slices or for a lower potassium option try strawberries, blueberries, or raspberries.

Nutrition Info

Calories 215
Carbohydrates 29 g
Protein 9 g
Dietary Fiber 6 g
Sodium 116 mg

24 Blueberry Whipped Pie

Prep/Cook Time: 7 mins
Serves: 9

Ingredients

- ~2 cups graham cracker crumbs
- 1 teaspoon cinnamon
- 1/2 cup unsalted butter, melted
- 8 ounces cream cheese, softened
- 1/4 cup granulated sugar
- 1 teaspoon vanilla extract
- 2 teaspoons lemon juice
- 8 ounce tub non dairy whipped cream
- 3 cups blueberries

Instructions

- Preheat oven to 375 degrees.
- In a medium bowl, combine the graham cracker crumbs, cinnamon, and melted butter.
- Press the mixture evenly into the bottom of a 9 inch round or square baking dish to form a crust.
- Bake crust for 7 minutes and let cool.
- In a large bowl, use an electric mixer to mix softened cream cheese with sugar until smooth.
- Mix in vanilla extract and lemon juice.
- Gently fold in the whipped topping then fold in the blueberries.
- Spread mixture evenly over the crust.
- Cover and chill in the refrigerator for at least 1 hour.

Nutrition Info

Calories 343
Carbohydrates 36 g
Protein 4 g
Sodium 197 mg

25 Broccoli Chicken Casserole

Prep/Cook Time: 1 hr 20 mins
Serves: 6

Ingredients

- 2-3 cups cooked broccoli
- 1 medium onion, chopped
- 2-3 chicken breast, diced
- 2 tablespoons butter or margarine
- 2 eggs, beaten
- 2 cups milk
- 2 cups cooked rice, barley, or noodles
- 2 cups grated cheese
- grated parmesan to top

Instructions

- Preheat oven to 350 degrees.
- Place broccoli in microwavable bowl, cover with plastic wrap and microwave until bright green, about 2-3 minutes.
- Meanwhile, brown onion and chicken in butter in a pan.

- Mix all ingredients and put in greased casserole dish.
- Sprinkle top with grated parmesan and bake about 1 hour and 15 minutes, until set and fork comes out clean.

Nutrition Info

Calories 368

Carbohydrates 26 g
Protein 26 g
Sodium 388 mg
Potassium 371 mg
Phosphorus 243 mg

26 Caramel Apple Pound Cake

Prep/Cook Time: 55 mins
Serves: 12

Ingredients

- 3 medium Granny Smith apples, peeled, cored and diced
- 1 box yellow cake mix or sugar free cake mix
- 3/4 cup flour
- 12 egg whites
- 1/4 cup vegetable oil
- 2 tablespoons water
- 1/4 cup caramel flavored syrup, regular or sugar free

Instructions

- Preheat oven to 350 degrees. Microwave diced apples for 6 minutes on high or until they are soft. Mash until applesauce and let cool to room temperature.
- In a mixing bowl add cake mix, flour, egg whites, vegetable oil, water, apple mixture and caramel flavoring. Mix on low speed for one minute, scraping the sides of the bowl. Then mix for 2 minutes on medium speed.
- Pour the batter into two greased loaf pans or a 9 X 13 baking dish. Bake for 30-45 minutes. The cake is done when a

toothpick stuck in the middle comes out clean. After the cake has cooled sprinkle with powdered sugar before serving.

Nutrition Info

Calories 300
Carbohydrates 52 g
Protein 7 g
Sodium 319 mg

27 Apple Cup Cider

Prep/Cook Time: 10 mins
Serves: 8

Ingredients

- 2 quarts 100% apple juice
- 2 cinnamon sticks
- 1/2 teaspoon cloves, whole
- 1 pinch nutmeg
- 1 teaspoon allspice

Instructions
- Pour apple juice into a large saucepan and begin heating over medium high heat.
- Add the rest of the ingredients.
- Bring to a boil, then reduce heat to low. Let "steep" for 10 minutes.
- When ready to serve, pour cider through a fine metal sieve into a mug or thermos.

Nutrition Info
Calories 114
Carbohydrates 28 g
Protein 0 g
Dietary Fiber 0 g
Fat 0 g
Sodium 28 mg

28 Beef Jerky

Serves: 30

Ingredients

- 3 pounds flank steak or other lean meat
- 3/4 cup sodium reduced (lite) soy sauce
- 1/2 cup red wine
- 1/4 cup dark brown sugar
- 2 tablespoons liquid smoke
- 1 1/2 teaspoons Worcestershire sauce
- 2-3 drops Tabasco sauce
- 1 teaspoon garlic powder
- 1 teaspoon liquid pepper sauce

Instructions

- Trim (or have the butcher trim) all fat from a 3 pound flank steak or any lean meat.
- Cut lengthwise, with the grain, into 30 long strips.
- Place the strips in a glass dish.
- mix all other ingredients together and pour over the beef.
- Cover and refrigerate for at least 5 hours or overnight.

- When you are ready to dry the meat, remove it from the marinade.
- If you have a dehydrator, set it for 145 degrees and dry the meat for 5-20 hours.
- If you are using the oven, preheat to 175 degrees.
- Put wire racks on top of baking sheets and lay the strips so they are not overlapping .
- Bake for 10-12 hours. The beef jerky should be dry and somewhat brittle when done.

Store your jerky in an airtight container or plastic bag. If you are keeping it for longer than a week, store it in the freezer.

Nutrition Info

Calories 100
Carbohydrates tbd
Protein 12 g
Sodium 100 mg
Potassium 100 mg
Phosphorus 190 mg

29 BBQ Winter Squash

Prep/Cook Time: 7 mins
Serves: 8

Ingredients

- 1-2 acorn or butternut squash sliced in 1" thick slices
- 1-2 tablespoons olive oil

- 1-2 tablespoons brown sugar
- 1-2 tablespoons butter

Instructions
- Heat grill until quite hot, (about 400 degrees).
- Brush squash with light coating of olive oil and place on grill about 5 minutes and turn.
- When fork tender, brush with melted butter and brown sugar.
- Leave on grill 1 minute, remove and serve.

Nutrition Info
Calories 99
Carbohydrates 19 g
Protein 1 g
Dietary Fiber 3 g
Sodium 6 mg
Potassium 508 mg
Phosphorus 53 mg

30 Mediterranean Green Beans

Prep/Cook Time: 6 mins
Serves 4

Ingredients

- 1 pound fresh green beans, trimmed to 1- to 2-inch pieces
- ¾ cup water
- 2 ½ teaspoons olive oil
- 3 fresh garlic cloves, minced

- 3 tablespoons fresh lemon juice
- 1/8 teaspoon ground black pepper

Instructions

- Bring water to a boil in large, nonstick skillet; add beans, cook 3 minutes; then drain and set aside.
- Heat skillet over medium-high heat and add oil; add garlic and beans; and sauté for 1 minute.
- Add juice and pepper and sauté 1 minute longer.

Nutrition Info

Calories 71 cal
Total Fat 3 g
Saturated Fat 0 g
Trans Fat 0 g
Cholesterol 0 mg
Sodium 2 mg
Carbohydrates 10 g
Protein 2 g

31 Banana-Apple Smoothie

Serves: 1

Ingredients

- 1/2 banana, peeled & cut into chunks
- 1/2 cup plain yogurt

- 1/2 cup unsweetened applesauce
- 1/4 cup skim milk
- 1 tablespoon honey
- 2 tablespoons oat bran

Instructions

- Place banana, yogurt, applesauce, milk, and honey in blender.
- Blend until smooth.
- Add oat bran and blend until thickened.

Nutrition Info
Calories 292
Carbohydrates 61 g
Protein 9 g
Sodium 103 mg
Potassium 609 mg
Phosphorus 140 mg

32 Basil Oil

Prep/Cook Time: 30 mins
Serves: 16

Ingredients

- 1 1/2 cups fresh basil leaves
- 1 cup olive oil or vegetable oil

Instructions

- Rinse and drain 1 1/2 cups lightly packed fresh basil leaves.
- Pat leaves dry with towel.
- In a blender or food processor, combine basil leaves and 1 cup olive oil or vegetable oil. Whirl just until leaves are finely chopped (do not puree).
- Pour mixture into a 1 to 1 1/2 quart pan over medium heat. Stir occasionally until oil bubbles around pan sides and reaches 165 degrees on a thermometer, 3-4 minutes. Be sure the oil is heated to this temperature to kill any bacteria in the mixture.
- Remove from heat and let stand until cool, about an hour.
- Line fine wire strainer with two layers of cheesecloth and set over a small bowl.
- Pour oil mixture into strainer.
- After oil passes through, gently press basil to remaining oil.
- Discard basil.
- Serve oil or store in an airtight container in the refrigerator up to 3 months. The olive oil may solidify slightly when chilled, but will quickly liquefy when it comes back to room temperature.

Nutrition Info

Calories 135
Carbohydrates 0 g
Protein 0 g
Dietary Fiber 15 g
Sodium 0 mg

33 Microwave Lemon Curd

Prep/Cook Time: 40 mins
Serves: 16

Ingredients

- 1 cup granulated sugar
- 3 eggs
- 2/3 cup fresh lemon juice
- 3 lemons, zested
- 1/2 cup butter, melted

Instructions

- In a microwave-safe bowl, whisk together the sugar & eggs until smooth.
- Stir in the lemon juice, lemon zest and butter.
- Cook in the microwave for one minute intervals, stirring after each minute until the mixture is thick enough to coat the back of a metal spoon.
- Remove from the microwave and pour into small sterile jars.
- Store for up to three weeks in the refrigerator.

Nutrition Info
Calories 115
Carbohydrates 14 g
Protein 1 g
Sodium 54 mg

34 Oven Fried Fish

Prep/Cook Time:
Serves: 4

Ingredients

- 1 1/2 tablespoons lemon juice
- 1 tablespoon olive oil
- 3 tablespoons Mrs. Dash Garlic & Herb Blend
- 1 1/2 tablespoons cumin
- 2 teaspoons Mrs. Dash Extra Spicy Blend
- 1/2 teaspoon grated lemon zest
- 1/3 cup corn meal
- 1 to 1 1/4 pounds catfish or other white fish filets

Instructions

- Preheat oven to 400 degrees.
- Combine lemon juice, olive oil, 1 Tbsp Mrs. Dash® Garlic & Herb, cumin and 1 tsp Mrs. Dash® Extra Spicy in a small container with lid.
- Shake well to blend ingredients.
- Pour mixture into shallow bowl; coat fish on both sides with lemon juice mixture.
- Combine corn meal, remaining Mrs. Dash® Seasoning Blends, and lemon rind. Mix to blend.
- Coat fish on both sides with corn meal mixture.
- Bake for 20 to 25 minutes or until fish flakes easily with a fork.
- Serve with additional lemon juice and hot pepper sauce, if desired.

Nutrition Info

Calories 264
Carbohydrates 13 g
Protein 20 g
Dietary Fiber 13 g
Fat 1 g
Sodium 67 mg
Potassium 526 mg

Phosphorus 230 mg

35 Paella

Prep/Cook Time: 20 mins
Serves: 6-8

Ingredients

Based on 6-8 servings per recipe.

- 1 tablespoon olive oil
- 1/2 pound Italian sausage
- 1/2 pound chicken breast, diced
- 1-2 garlic cloves, pressed
- 2 cups uncooked short grain rice
- 1 cup yellow onion, chopped
- 1 1/2 cups low sodium chicken broth
- 2 jars roasted red peppers, pureed
- 1/2 teaspoon paprika
- 1/2 teaspoon Tabasco sauce
- 10 strands or 1/8 teaspoon saffron
- 1/2 pound shrimp, uncooked, shelled, deveined
- 1/2 cup each red & green peppers, sliced in strips
- 1/2 cup frozen green peas

Instructions

- Heat olive oil in large pan and saute sausage, chicken, and garlic until meat is browned.
- Remove meats and set aside.

- Add rice and onion to pan and saute until onion is translucent and rice is golden brown.
- Add meat back to pan with broth and pureed red bell peppers.
- Add paprika, Tabasco, and saffron.
- Bring to a boil; reduce heat to low, and simmer covered for 10 minutes.
- Stir in shrimp, bell peppers, and peas.
- Cover and cook 10 minutes.

Nutrition Info

Calories 233
Carbohydrates 25 g
Protein 20 g
Dietary Fiber 6 g
Fat 2 g
Sodium 257 mg
Potassium 330 mg
Phosphorus 201 mg

36 Parslied Onions and Pinto Beans

Serves: 8-12

Ingredients

- 1 cup Italian parsley, flat-leafed
- 1 cup curly parsley
- 1/2 cup fresh dill
- 1 large lemon
- 2 cups low salt chicken broth

- 2 tablespoons butter
- 1 tablespoon oil
- 6 cups onions, sliced
- 1/2 teaspoon curry powder
- 4 cups pinto beans, low sodium
- to taste pepper

Instructions

- Wash and dry the parsley and dill.
- Remove any thick stems and chop into 1/2 – 1 inch pieces; set aside.
- Halve the lemon and squeeze the juice; set aside.
- Put the halved lemon and broth in a small saucepan.
- Bring the broth to a boil, lower heat, and simmer, covered.
- In a large saucepan, heat the butter and oil and cook the onions until wilted and golden.
- Stir in the curry powder, parsley, and dill.
- Add the broth and lemon halves.
- Cook slowly to tenderize the parsley and slightly reduce the broth. (If you cover the pan, the parsley loses some of its brilliant color.)
- Stir in the beans and the lemon juice and heat through.
- Remove lemon halves.
- Season with pepper.

Nutrition Info

Calories 458
Carbohydrates 78 g
Protein 26 g
Sodium 140 mg
Potassium 207 mg
Phosphorus 432 mg

37 Mediterranean Pizza

Prep/Cook Time: 20 mins
Serves: 12

Ingredients

- 1 crust, 2 pitas ready made pizza dough or large pitas
- 1 tablespoon olive oil
- 2 garlic cloves, sliced thinly
- 1 roma tomato, sliced
- 10 basil leaves, thinly sliced
- 3 ounces goat cheese, or ricotta

Instructions

- Preheat oven to 450 degrees.
- Coat pizza crust with olive oil.
- Arrange garlic slices evenly across the crust.
- Cover garlic with tomato slices.
- Sprinkle basil evenly over pizza then top with goat cheese.
- Bake in oven for 10-15 minutes or as otherwise directed by crust package intructions.

Nutrition Info

Calories 176
Carbohydrates 18 g
Protein 7 g
Dietary Fiber 8 g
Fat 0 g

Sodium 240 mg
Potassium 86 g
Phosphorus 90 g

38 Master Mix

Prep/Cook Time: 10 mins
Serves: 13 cups

Ingredients

- 8 1/2 cups all-purpose flour
- 1 tablespoon baking powder
- 2 teaspoons cream of tartar
- 1 teaspoon baking soda
- 1 1/2 cups instant nonfat milk powder
- 2 1/4 cups vegetable shortening

Instructions

- Sift together flour, baking powder, cream of tartar, baking soda, and milk powder.
- Cut in shortening with a pastry blender until evenly distributed.
- Store in a large, airtight container in a cool, dry place.
- Use within 10-12 weeks.

Nutrition Info

Calories 640
Carbohydrates 67 g

Protein 11 g
Dietary Fiber 36 g
Sodium 271 mg
Potassium 298 mg
Phosphorus 189 mg

39 Mediterranean Lamb Patties

Prep/Cook Time: 10 mins
Serves: 4

Ingredients

- 1 lb. ground lamb
- 1 whole egg
- 1/4 cup panko* bread crumbs
- 1/4 cup onion, finely chopped
- 1 clove garlic, finely chopped
- 1 teaspoon dried oregano (or dried mint)
- 1/2 teaspoon ground pepper
- 1/2 cup feta cheese, crumbled

Instructions

- In a large bowl, combine all ingredients, mixing well.
- Form into four equal sized patties, about 1/2 inch thick.
- Preheat a large non-stick skillet over medium-high heat.
- Add patties and keep the heat high until browned, then flip, about 5 minutes each side and turn down the heat.

- Be sure patties are cooked all the way through, no longer pink in the middle or when internal temperature reaches 160 degrees.

Nutrition Info

Calories 305
Carbohydrates 5 g
Protein 19 g
Sodium 229 mg
Potassium 45 mg
Phosphorus 74 mg

40 Oven Fried Chicken

Prep/Cook Time: 1 hr, 10 mins
Serves: 8

Ingredients

- 1/4 cup butter
- 1/4 cup corn oil
- 1/2 cup flour
- 1/2 cup cornmeal
- 1 tablespoon paprika
- 1 teaspoon ground pepper
- 1 teaspoon ground mustard
- 1 tablespoon dried tarragon
- 1 tablespoon dried marjoram
- 4 pounds whole chicken, cut up into pieces

Instructions

- Heat oven to 425 degrees.
- Put 1/4 cup butter and 1/4 cup oil in bottom of 9×13 inch pan.
- Put pan in oven to melt butter and oil.
- While butter and oil mixture is melting, put 1/2 cup flour and 1/2 cup cornmeal in a big zip lock plastic bag.
- Add seasonings.
- Drop in chicken pieces and shake
- Lay chicken pieces, skin side down, in hot oil in pan.
- Bake 30 minutes.
- Turn over and bake about 20-30 minutes more (smaller pieces like thighs and gizzards may take less time).

Nutrition Info

Calories 376
Carbohydrates 15 g
Protein 24 g
Dietary Fiber 24 g
Sodium 109 mg

41 Pancit Guisado

Prep/Cook Time: 25 mins
Serves: 6

Ingredients

- 8 ounces rice stick noodles (bihon)
- 1/4 cup vegetable oil

- 3 cloves garlic, minced
- 1/2 medium onion, chopped
- 1 pound chicken breast or pork, boiled & sliced
- 1 1/2 cups shredded green cabbage
- 1 large carrot, peeled & cut like matchsticks
- 1 tablespoon reduced sodium soy sauce
- 1 cup low sodium chicken broth
- 1 stalk celery, sliced
- 2 green onions, chopped
- 1 lemon (optional)

Instructions

- Soak rice noodles in warm water for 5 minutes, drain and set aside.
- Heat oil in a large skillet or wok over medium heat.
- Add garlic and onion and saute for 5 minutes.
- Add sliced meat, cabbage, and carrots.
- Stir- fry for 3 minutes.
- Add reduced sodium soy sauce, chicken broth, and celery.
- Simmer for 3 minutes.
- Add soaked rice noodles to broth and simmer for 3 minutes.
- Top noodles with meat and vegetable mixture, garnish with green onions and flavor with fresh squeezed lemon juice, if desired.

Nutrition Info

Calories 287
Carbohydrates 39 g
Protein 19 g
Sodium 194 mg
Potassium 391 mg
Phosphorus 183 m

42 Berry Wild Rice Salad

Prep/Cook Time: 55 mins
Serves: 8-10

Ingredients

- 1 cup uncooked wild rice
- 2 cups water
- 1 cup collard greens, lightly steamed
- 1/2 cup onion, chopped
- 2 1/2 cups mixed berries (raspberry, blackberry, etc)
- 1/4 cup blueberries
- 2 tablespoons lemon juice
- 1/4 cup fresh mint, chopped
- 1 tablespoon olive oil
- 1/2 cup fat free or reduced fat sour cream

Instructions

- Place rice and water in a large saucepan.
- Bring to a boil, reduce heat to low and simmer covered for about 45-55 minutes, or until most of the liquid is absorbed.
- Empty rice into a large mixing bowl and add steamed greens, onion, and berries.
- Mix well.
- In a blender or food processor, puree all dressing ingredients except sour cream until it is well blended, adding more liquid if necessary.
- Slowly whisk in sour cream until well mixed.
- Pour dressing over rice salad and toss to coat.

- Serve immediately or store covered in the refrigerator for later use.

Nutrition Info

Calories 133
Carbohydrates 25 g
Protein 4 g
Dietary Fiber 2 g
Fat 4 g
Sodium 26 mg
Potassium 159 mg
Phosphorus 111 mg

43 Low Salt Stir-Fry

Prep/Cook Time: 15 mins
Serves: 2

Ingredients

- 4 cups (about 3/4 pound) mixed greens (lettuce,collard, beet, etc)
- 1 tablespoon olive oil
- 1 cup onions, sliced thin
- 1/4 teaspoon curry powder
- 1 tablespoon low sodium soy sauce
- 1/2 cup white wine vinegar or rice vinegar
- 8 ounces tofu, cut into cubes
- 1/2 teaspoon sesame oil
- 1/2 teaspoon sesame seeds

Instructions

- Cut greens into 2 inch long shreds.
- Heat oil in wok or saute pan.
- Saute onions until translucent, about 2 minutes.
- Sprinkle curry over onions and add sugar and greens.
- Cover.
- Reduce heat and let greens steam in their own juice until tender, 5-8 minutes. (During this time, uncover and turn occasionally. Add a little water if sticking.) Don't overcook or greens will turn darker.
- Remove greens with slotted spoon leaving juices in pan.
- Add soy sauce and vinegar, heat to boiling.
- When sauce is slightly thickened, remove from heat and poor over greens.
- Garnish with sesame oil and seeds.

Nutrition Info

Calories 231
Carbohydrates 13 g
Protein 14 g
Sodium 355 mg
Potassium 442 mg
Phosphorus 54 mg

44 Beef or Chicken Enchiladas

Prep/Cook Time: 20 mins
Serves: 5

Ingredients

- 1 pound lean ground beef or chicken
- 1/2 cup onion, chopped
- 1 teaspoon cumin
- 1/2 teaspoon black pepper
- 1 garlic clove, chopped
- 12 corn tortillas
- 1 can enchilada sauce

Instructions

- Preheat oven to 375 degrees.
- Brown meat in frying pan.
- Add onion, garlic, cumin and pepper. Continue cooking. Stir until onions are soft.
- In another pan fry tortillas in a small amout of oil.
- Dip each tortilla in enchilada sauce.
- Fill with meat mixture and roll up.
- Place enchilada in a shallow pan and top with sauce and cheese if desired.
- Bake until cheese is melted and enchiladas are golden brown.

- Served with sour cream, sliced olives, or other topping of your choice.

Nutrition Info

Calories 235
Carbohydrates 30
Protein 13 g
Dietary Fiber 14 g
Sodium 201 mg

45 Mexican Brunch Eggs

Prep/Cook Time: 1 hr, 10 mins
Serves: 8

Ingredients

- 1/2 cup chopped onion
- 2 cloves garlic, crushed
- 2 tablespoons margarine
- 1 1/2 cups frozen corn, thawed
- 1 1/2 teaspoons ground cumin
- 1/8 teaspoon cayenne pepper
- 8 eggs, beaten
- 8 slices toasted bread

Instructions

- In a large skillet, saute onion and garlic in margarine until onion is soft.
- Add corn, cumin, and cayenne; stir to combine.
- Pour in eggs or egg substitute and cook over low heat, stirring occasionally until eggs are set.
- Arrange toast triangles on a large platter.
- Spoon egg mixture on toast triangles.
- Serve immediately.

Nutrition Info

Calories 214
Carbohydrates 13 g
Protein 9 g

Dietary Fiber 14 g
Sodium 147 mg

46 Black-Eyed Peas

Prep/Cook Time: 1 hr, 40 mins
Serves: 12

Ingredients

- 2 cups Black-eyed peas, soaked overnight
- 3 1/2 cups water or low-sodium vegetable stock
- 12 ounces smoked turkey (optional)
- 1 medium onion, finely chopped
- 5 to 6 cloves garlic, finely chopped
- 1 cup celery, diced
- 1/2 teaspoon thyme
- 1/2 teaspoon ginger
- 1/2 teaspoon curry powder
- 1 pinch cayenne pepper

Instructions

- Place black-eyed peas and liquid in large pot with vegetables, seasonings and meat (optional).
- Bring to a boil, then reduce heat to low, cover with a lid and cook until peas are tender, which will take about 1 1/2 hours.
- Stir occasionally.

Nutrition Info

Calories 130
Carbohydrates 19 g
Protein 12 g
Dietary Fiber 1 g
Sodium 274 mg
Potassium 434 mg
Phosphorus 200 mg

47 Pancakes with Master Mix

Prep/Cook Time: 15 mins
Serves: 5

Ingredients

- 2 1/4 cups Master Mix
- 1 tablespoon sugar
- 1 egg, beaten
- 1 1/2 cups milk

Instructions
- Combine Master Mix and sugar in a medium bowl.
- Combine egg and milk in a small bowl and add all at once to dry ingredients.
- Blend well.
- Let stand for 5-10 minutes.
- Cook on a hot oiled grill about 3-4 minutes or until browned on both sides.
Nutrition Info

Calories 348
Carbohydrates 36 g
Protein 9 g
Dietary Fiber 19 g
Sodium 302 mg
Potassium 260 mg
Phosphorus 175 mg

48 Berrylicious Smoothie

Prep/Cook Time: 10 mins
Serves: 2

Ingredients

- 1/4 cup cranberry juice cocktail
- 2/3 cup silken tofu, firm
- 1/2 cup raspberries, frozen, unsweetened
- 1/2 cup blueberries, frozen, unsweetened
- 1 teaspoon vanilla extract
- 1/2 teaspoon powdered lemonade, such as Country Time

Instructions

- Pour juice into a blender.
- Add rest of ingredients.
- Blend until very smooth.
- Serve immediately and enjoy!

Nutrition Info
Calories 115

Carbohydrates 18 g
Protein 6 g
Dietary Fiber 1 g
Fat 3 g

49 Irish Baked Potato Soup

Prep/Cook Time: 1 hr 30 mins
Serves: 6

Ingredients

- 2 large potatoes (russetts work best)
- 1/3 cup flour
- 4 cups skim milk
- 1/2 teaspoon pepper
- 4 ounces cheese, cubed
- 1/2 cup fat free sour cream

Instructions

- Bake potatoes at 400 degrees until tender or in microwave until done.
- Let cool and cut lengthwise and scoop out pulp.
- On medium heat, brown flour to a light brown color and gradually add milk, stirring until well blended.
- Add potato pulp and pepper.
- Cook over medium heat until thick and bubbly, stirring frequently.
- Add cheese, stir until melted.

- Remove from heat and stir in sour cream.

Nutrition Info

Calories 275
Carbohydrates 39 g
Protein 14 g
Dietary Fiber 7 g
Sodium 226 mg

50 Italian Meatballs

Prep/Cook Time: 20 mins
Serves: 12

Ingredients

- 1.5 pounds ground beef
- 2 large eggs, beaten
- 1/2 cup dry oatmeal flakes
- 3 tablespoons parmesan cheese
- 1/2 tablespoon olive oil
- 1/2 tablespoon garlic powder
- 1 teaspoon dried oregano
- 1/2 cup onion, chopped
- 1/2 teaspoon black pepper

Instructions

- Preheat oven to 375 degrees.
- Combine all ingredients in a large bowl and mix together.

- Roll into 1" balls and place on a baking sheet.
- Bake for 10 to 15 minutes, until meatballs are cooked through.
- To serve, place meatballs in a warming dish or crock pot on low heat setting. Serve with 2 teaspoons sauce on the side.

Nutrition Info

Calories 163
Carbohydrates 4 g
Protein 13 g
Sodium 72 mg

51 Jammin' Jambalaya

Prep/Cook Time: 40 mins
Serves: 6

Ingredients

- 2 teaspoons olive oil
- 1/2 pound jumbo shrimp, cooked, tails removed
- 7 ounces smoked turkey sausage, sliced
- 1/2 large yellow onion, chopped
- 1 large red bell pepper, chopped
- 3 cups collard greens, chopped
- 2 garlic cloves, minced
- 1/4 teaspoon cayenne pepper
- 1/8 teaspoon white pepper
- 1/4 teaspoon black pepper
- 1/2 teaspoon dry thyme or 1-2 teaspoons fresh thyme
- 1/2 teaspoon oregano

- 2 bay leaves
- 1/4 teaspoon allspice
- 1/2 cup rice (white or brown)
- 1 2/3 cups chicken broth

Instructions

- Heat olive oil in a large skillet over medium-high heat.
- Add shrimp, turkey sausage, onion, bell pepper, collards and garlic.
- Cook for 10 minutes, stirring occasionally.
- Add remaining ingredients and bring to a boil.
- Cover, reduce heat to medium-low and simmer for 20 minutes or until rice is tender. (35-40 if using brown rice).

Nutrition Info

Calories 200
Carbohydrates 19 g
Protein 16 g
Dietary Fiber 6 g
Fat 2 g

52 Bran Breakfast Bars

Prep/Cook Time: 45 mins
Serves: 12

Ingredients

- 1 cup boiling water
- 1/3 cup chopped raisins or med. dates, diced

- 1 cup oatmeal
- 1/2 cup whole wheat flour
- 1/3 cup oil (corn, soybean, or safflower)
- 1 1/2 cups pure bran
- 3 tablespoons brown-type granular sugar substitute

Instructions

- Pour boiling water over diced fruit.
- Allow to stand at least 20 minutes.
- Combine dry ingredients in a large mixing bowl.
- Drain fruit, adding boiling water to the drained liquid to make 1 cup and put in blender with oil.
- Blend 1 minute.
- Immediately pour into dry ingredients and mix well.
- Add fruit and remix.
- Place batter in non-stick 8"x10" baking dish.
- Level with fingers or spatula and then mark cuttings: 4 rows the narrow way and 6 rows the long way.
- Bake in a preheated oven at 375F for 22 minutes.
- Cool on rack.
- Refrigerate or freeze if keeping more than 2 days.

Nutrition Info

Calories 158
Carbohydrates 24 g
Protein 4 g
Sodium 2 mg

53 Mediterranean Roasted Red Pepper Soup

Prep/Cook Time: 35 mins

Serves: 6

Ingredients

- 2 tablespoons olive oil
- 2 large onions, diced
- 6 garlic cloves, minced
- 1 teaspoon paprika
- 1/2 cup lentils, rinsed and sorted
- 3 fresh red peppers, roasted
- 1 (28 ounce) can diced tomatoes
- 2 cups low sodium chicken broth or water
- 2/3 cup nonfat dry milk
- 1 tablespoon red wine vinegar
- 1/4 cup cashews or almonds, toasted

Instructions

- Heat olive oil, add onions and cook slowly, stirring occasionally until onions are very soft and carmelized.
- Add garlic and paprika, cook for 2 minutes.
- Add lentils, peppers, tomatoes, and 1 cup broth.
- Bring to boil, reduce heat to maintain a steady simmer, cover, and cook lentils until they are soft (about 30 min).
- In several batches, whirl soup in blender or food processor until very smooth.
- Add dry milk and vinegar to the last batch.
- Stir together.
- Season with more vinegar if needs more taste and add in a little more broth if soup seems too thick.
- Serve topped with a sparkle of almonds or cashews and a drizzle of oil if you like.

Nutrition Info

Calories 240
Carbohydrates 31 g
Protein 11 g
Dietary Fiber 9 g
Sodium 128 mg

54 Low Salt Ketchup

Serves: 64

Ingredients

- 3/4 cup onion, chopped
- 1/2 cup cider vinegar
- 1/3 cup sugar
- 1 tablespoon molasses
- 2 teaspoons dry mustard
- 1/2 teaspoon celery seed
- 1/4 teaspoon ground cinnamon
- 1/4 teaspoon cloves
- 1/4 teaspoon dried basil
- 1/4 teaspoon dried tarragon
- 1/4 teaspoon pepper
- 1 clove garlic, minced
- 1 cup water
- 2 (6-oz.) can tomato paste

Instructions

- Place all ingredients except water and tomato paste in a blender or food processor, blend until smooth.
- Pour mixture into a Dutch oven or large sauce pan.
- Stir in 3 cups water and two 6-oz. cans tomato paste.
- Simmer, uncovered, about 35 minutes or until mixture is reduced to half its original amount, stirring occasionally.
- Pour into jars and store in refrigerator for up to 1 month. Or pour into 1-cup freezer containers; seal, label, and freeze for up to 10 months. Makes 5 cups.

Nutrition Info

Calories 12
Carbohydrates 3 g
Protein 0 g
Sodium 17 mg

55 Master Ground Beef Mix

Serves: 8

Ingredients

- 2 pounds ground beef
- 1 cup diced onion
- 3 tablespoons Worcestershire sauce
- 1 teaspoon Italian seasoning
- 1 teaspoon garlic powder

- 1/4 teaspoon pepper
- 4 slices white bread, cubed
- 1/2 cup milk

Instructions

- In a large fry pan, on the stove top, mix all ingredients.
- Cook, stirring occasionally, until meat is no longer red.
- Remove meat from heat, drain excess liquid.
- Let cool in the refrigerator.
- Portion 1 cup meat in to freeze containers or freezer weight bags.
- Freeze for later use in tacos, Shepard's pie, nachos, stroganoff, goulash, soups, or casseroles.
- Keeps for 3 months in the freezer

Nutrition Info

Calories 331
Carbohydrates 13 g
Protein 32 g
Sodium 215 mg

56 Microwave Berry Jam

Prep/Cook Time: 20 mins
Serves: 16

Ingredients

- 1 cup mashed berries (any kind or combination)
- 3/4 cup granulated sugar
- 1/4 teaspoon unsalted butter
- 1 teaspoon lemon juice

Instructions

- Put ingredients in a microwave proof bowl and mix.
- Microwave on high for 5 minutes for all berries except strawberries, which should be microwaved for 4 minutes.
- Stir.
- Microwave another 5 minutes, (4 for Strawberries).
- Put in container with lid or cover with plastic wrap, keep refrigerated.
- Keeps for several months.

Nutrition Info

Calories 41
Carbohydrates 10 g
Protein 0 g
Dietary Fiber 0 g
Fat 0 g

57 Apple Filled Crepes

Serves: 1 crepe

Ingredients

- 4 egg yolks
- 2 whole eggs
- 1/2 cup sugar
- 1 cup flour
- 1/4 cup oil
- 2 cups milk
- 4 apples
- 1/2 cup brown sugar

- 1/2 teaspoon cinnamon
- 1/2 teaspoon nutmeg
- 1 stick or 1/2 cup unsalted butter

Instructions

- Mix egg yolks, whole eggs, sugar, flour, oil, and milk until the batter is free of lumps.
- Heat a small non-stick skillet over medium heat.
- Spray pan with cooking spray.
- Using a 2 ounce ladle or 1/4 cup, spoon 1 scoop of batter into the pan, then swirl the pan to spread the crepe batter thinly on the bottom of the pan.
- Cook for about 20 seconds, then flip the crepe (with the aid of a rubber spatula) and cook for about 10 seconds. Set crepes aside while you make the filling.
- Peel, core, and slice apples each into 12 slices.
- Heat a medium saute pan.
- Melt butter, then add brown sugar.
- Toss in the apples, cinnamon, and nutmeg.
- Cook apples until tender but not mushy. Set aside to cool.
- Assembling the Crepes: Fill the middle of each crepe about with about 2 tablespoons of apple filling.
- Roll into a log.

Note: Crepes can be made the day before or hours in advance, just cover with plastic wrap and store in the refrigerator. When ready to eat microwave crepes for a few seconds.

Nutrition Info

Calories 315
Carbohydrates 40 g
Protein 5 g
Dietary Fiber 15 g

58 Banana Oat Shake

Prep/Cook Time: 20 mins
Serves: 2

Ingredients

- 1/2 cup cooked oatmeal, chilled
- 2/3 cup skim milk
- 2 tablespoons brown sugar
- 1 tablespoon wheat germ
- 1 1/2 teaspoons vanilla extract
- 1/2 frozen banana, cut into chunks

Instructions

- Place oatmeal in blender and blend for a few minutes.
- Add milk, brown sugar, wheat germ, vanilla, and 1/2 banana. Blend until thick and smooth.

Nutrition Info

Calories 172
Carbohydrates 33 g
Protein 6 g
Sodium 42 mg

59 Baked Potato Soup

Prep/Cook Time: 30 mins
Serves: 6

Ingredients

- 2 large potatoes
- 1/3 cup flour
- 4 cups skim milk
- 1/2 teaspoon pepper
- 4 ounces, shredded reduce fat monterey jack cheese
- 1/2 cup fat free sour cream

Instructions

- Bake potatoes at 400 degrees until fork tender.
- Let cool.
- Cut lengthwise and scoop out pulp.
- Place flour in large sauce pan. Gradually add milk, stirring until blended.
- Add potato pulp and pepper.
- Cook over medium heat until thick and bubbly, stirring frequently.
- Add cheese, stir until cheese melts.
- Remove from heat and stir in sour cream.

Nutrition Info

Calories 216
Carbohydrates 29 g
Protein 15 g
Dietary Fiber 4 g
Fat 1 g

60 Apple and Cream Cheese Torte

Prep/Cook Time: 1 hr, 5 min
Serves: 10

Ingredients

- 1/2 cup unsalted butter, softened
- 3/4 cup sugar, divided in 1/4 cups
- 1 cup flour
- 8 ounces cream cheese, softened
- 1 egg
- 1 teaspoon vanilla
- 3-4 medium apples, thinly sliced
- 1/2 teaspoon cinnamon

Instructions

- Preheat oven to 450 degrees.
- In a medium bowl, cream butter and 1/4 cup of sugar.
- Blend in flour.
- Press into a spring form pan.
- Beat cream cheese, 1/4 cup of sugar, egg, and vanilla until smooth.
- Spread into the spring form pan.
- Toss apples with remaining 1/4 cup of sugar and cinnamon.
- Arrange apples over cheese filling.
- Bake for 10 minutes.

- Reduce oven temperature to 400 degrees and bake for an additional 25-30 minutes until filling is firm and the apples have softened.

Nutrition Info

Calories 298
Carbohydrates 36 g
Protein 4 g
Sodium 176 mg

61 Orange Creamsicle Smoothie

Prep Time 5 minutes
Total Time 5 minutes
Servings: 2

Ingredients

- 2 oranges
- 2 bananas
- 1/4 cup almond milk or milk of your choice, 60 ml
- 1 teaspoon vanilla extract
- 1 cup crushed ice

Instructions

- Add everything to a blender or food processor and blend until smooth. For a thinner consistency add more almond milk and for a thicker consistency add more ice.

Nutrition Info

Calories: 176 Sodium: 47mg Carbohydrates: 42g Fiber: 6g Sugar: 26g Protein: 2g

62 Thai green curry

Prep Time 10 minutes
Cook Time 25 minutes
Total Time 35 minutes
Servings: 5

Ingredients

Curry Paste

- 2 stalks lemon grass
- 3-4 green chilis (depending on how much spice you can handle, deseed*
- 6 spring onions, green part only for low FODMAP
- 1 tablespoon fresh grated ginger or galangal
- 1/2 cup chopped fresh coriander/cilantro leaves & stems
- 1/2 cup fresh basil
- 1 teaspoon ground coriander
- 1 teapoon ground cumin
- 1 teaspoon fish sauce
- zest from one lime and half it's juice
- 1/2 teaspoon ground black pepper
- 2 tablespoon coconut oil

Chicken Curry

- 1.2 lb / 600g chicken breasts, or thigh fillets, cut into bite size pieces
- 1 can coconut milk 14oz/400g
- 1/2 cup chicken stock or water, 120 ml
- 1-2 teaspoons fish sauce, adjust for saltiness
- 2 sweet peppers, cut into strips
- 3/4 cup baby corn, 100 grams
- small handful spring onions cut into strips

Instructions

- Thinly slice the lemon grass stalks before adding it to a food processor with the remaining curry paste ingredients. Whiz everything together until you end up with a thick, green paste. You will probably need to stop every now and then to push the sides down with a spoon to get everything to blend properly. If you don't have a food processor you can also use a high powered blender, it may just take a little longer.
- Add the curry paste to a large pan and warm on a low heat for 2-3 minutes.
- Add the chicken to pan and stir, coating it in the curry paste. Cook for another 4-5 minutes on a medium heat. Add the coconut milk, chicken stock and fish sauce and bring to a boil for a couple of minutes.
- Turn the heat down, add the sweet peppers, baby corn, and spring onions and allow the curry to simmer for at least 15 minutes until the sauce thickens.
- Serve over rice to keep this low FODMAP, or cauliflower rice for a paleo option. Garnish with fresh basil/cilantro and add an extra squeeze of lemon juice for more brightness.

Nutrition Info

Calories: 400 Saturated Fat: 20g Cholesterol: 69mg Sodium: 419mg Carbohydrates: 16g Fiber: 2g Sugar: 4g Protein: 27g

63 Buckwheat & Oat Pancakes

Sweet and nutty aquafaba Buckwheat & Oat Pancakes - free from gluten, dairy, eggs, and refined sugar.

Prep Time 10 minutes
Cook Time 20 minutes
Total Time 30 minutes
Servings: 8

Ingredients

- 1 cup buckwheat flour
- 1 cup oat flour
- 2 1/2 teaspoons baking powder
- 1 teaspoon cinnamon
- 1/4 teaspoon sea salt
- 6 tablespoons aquafaba*
- 3 tablespoons maple syrup
- 1 1/2 cup dairy free buttermilk, see notes below for how to make
- 1 teaspoon vanilla extract
- coconut oil for frying pancakes

Instructions

- In a medium sized mixing bowl mix together the flours, baking powder, cinnamon, and sea salt and whisk to combine.
- In a liquid measuring cup add the buttermilk, aquafaba, maple syrup, and vanilla and whisk to combine.
- Pour the wet ingredients into the dry ingredients and whisk together. It's ok the leave a few lumps in the batter. You might notice that the batter starts to bubble slightly in places.
- Heat your skillet or griddle to a medium low heat and grease with a little bit of coconut oil. When the oil is hot, use a 1/4 cup measuring cup to pour the batter on the skillet. Cook for 2-3 minutes or until you notice little bubbles starting to form on the surface of the pancakes. Flip and cook for another 1-2 minutes on the other side.
- Transfer your cooked pancakes to a plate and continue the process until you're done. Make sure to add more coconut oil as needed.

Nutrition Info

Calories: 179

64 Homemade Gluten Free Flour Blend

Prep Time 5 minutes
Total Time 5 minutes
Servings: 3

Ingredients

- 1 1/4 cups White Rice Flour 180 grams
- 3/4 cups Brown Rice Flour |120 grams
- 2/3 cup Potato Starch | 112 grams
- 1/3 cup Tapioca Starch | 42 grams

Instructions

- Add all your flours to a bowl and whisk together. Take the time to fully blend everything together evenly. You can also toss your flours to a blender/food processor to blend.
- Store in an airtight jar/container.

Nutrition Info

Calories: 514 Carbohydrates: 118g Fiber: 2g Protein: 7g

65 Chicken Avocado & Raspberry Salad

Prep Time 10 minutes
Cook Time 5 minutes
Total Time 15 minutes
Servings: 4

Ingredients

Salad

- 3 cups salad greens of your choice, (I used a head of gem lettuce)
- 2 cooked, , skinless chicken breasts, chopped
- 6 slices pancetta, (can sub with streaky bacon slices)

- 1 cup raspberries
- 1 avocado, , sliced* see notes about fodmaps
- 1/4 cup chopped almonds

  Dressing

- 3 tablespoons fresh squeezed lemon juice
- 2 tablespoons maple syrup
- 2 teaspoons Dijon mustard
- 1 teaspoon whole grain mustard
- ¼ cup olive oil
- Salt and pepper to taste

Instructions

- Start by cooking the pancetta. Dry fry the slices in a medium sized skillet on a medium heat for a couple minutes on each side or until crispy. Once cooked remove from the heat and cool on a paper towel lined plate.
- Prep the salad by tossing together the rest of the salad ingredients in a large bowl. Once the pancetta is cool enough to handle break the slices into small pieces and scatter over the top of the salad.
- Make the dressing by adding all of the ingredients to a small jar with a lid. Close and shake until mixed and slightly emulsified.
- Drizzle the dressing over the top. You will end up with left over dressing (unless you really like salads doused in dressing).

Nutrition Info

Calories: 441 Saturated Fat: 6g Cholesterol: 61mg Sodium: 280mg Carbohydrates: 16g Fiber: 5g Sugar: 8g Protein: 21

66 No Bake Snickers Cheesecake (Vegan & Paleo)

Prep Time 30 minutes
Cook Time 5 minutes
Total Time 35 minutes
Servings: 16

Ingredients

CRUST

- 1 1/2 cup packed dates
- 1 1/2 cups raw pecans or walnuts

CHEESECAKE FILLING

- 2 cups raw cashews
- 1/2 cup full fat coconut milk
- 2 tablespoons maple syrup
- 1 teaspoon vanilla extract
- 3 tablespoon coconut oil
- 1 tablespoon lemon juice

NUT BUTTER CARAMEL

- 2 tablespoon maple syrup
- 2 tablespoon melted coconut oil
- 2 tablespoon peanut butter, or almond butter for paleo
- 1/2 teaspoon vanilla extract

TOPPINGS

- 1/2 cup salted peanuts or almonds for paleo
- 1/2 cup melted dark chocolate

Instructions

- If you haven't already add the cashews to a bowl and cover with water. Leave the cashews overnight to use when you need it the next day.

Crust

- Make the crust by adding the dates and the pecans to a food processor or high powered blender. Blitz together until the dates and pecans are broken up into small pieces and come together. If your mixture is too dry add a couple more dates. You may need to stop to scrape the sides down occasionally.
- Press the crust into an 8in x 8in parchment-lined dish, until evenly spread. Use another sheet of parchment paper to place over the crust when pressing in the pan. This will keep the crust from sticking to your hands when you're trying to press it into the tin.

Nut Butter Carame

- In a small pot melt the caramel ingredients on a medium low heat for about 2 minutes (the maple, oil, nut butter butter, vanilla, and sea salt). Make sure to stir while everything melts to keep from burning. Pour the caramel mixture into a small bowl so that it cools faster. Set it aside in the fridge while you make the filling.

Filling

- For the cheesecake layer, begin by draining the water from the cashews and then placing them in a high speed blender or food processor with the remaining cheesecake ingredients. Blend it all together until it becomes smooth. If you need, stop and scrap the sides down to get all the bits mixed in. This should take 60-90 seconds. (If you own a Blendtec, I put mine on the smoothie setting and that did the trick
- Taste and adjust flavor as needed. Add another 1-2 tablespoons of maple if you like it sweet. Keep in mind that the nut butter caramel will add additional sweetness when we add it in later.
- Pour filling over the crust. Dollop half of the caramel mixture across the cheesecake filling and then drag a knife or toothpick across the top to create the rippled effect. Don't worry if it's not pretty because you're going to later drizzle dark chocolate and the remaining caramel over the top of the cheesecake. Take half of the peanuts (or almonds) and scatter them across the pan and press them into the filling
- Cover the cheesecake and place it in the freezer for 4-5 hours to set.
- Remove the cheesecake from the freezer to allow it to thaw slightly before cutting it.
- While it's thawing melt your dark chocolate in the microwave in 30 second increments or over the stove top over a pot of simmering water on a low heat stirring constantly. Remove the chocolate from the heat and let it cool for a minute or two before drizzling it over the cheesecake.
- Drizzle the remaining nut butter caramel over the top along with the melted chocolate and remaining peanuts (or almonds).

Nutrition Info

Calories: 326 Saturated Fat: 9g Sodium: 38mg Carbohydrates: 24g Fiber: 3g Sugar: 15g Protein: 6g

67 Vegan Chocolate Caramel Turtle Clusters

Prep Time 45 minutes
Cook Time 10 minutes
Total Time 55 minutes
Servings: 20

Ingredients

Caramel

- 2 tablespoons |30 grams coconut oil
- 1/4 cup | 80 grams maple syrup
- 1/2 cup | 120 grams almond butter or peanut butter
- 1 teaspoon vanilla extract
- 1/4 teaspoon sea salt

Everything else

- 2 cups | 200 grams raw pecan halves
- 6 ounces | 175 grams dairy free chocolate chips, chopped or in chips

Instructions

- Preheat the oven to 350°F/180°C.
- Add all of the caramel ingredients to a small sauce pan and warm on a low heat. Stir together until the coconut oil and

the nut butter melts, then remove from the heat. Keep stirring until everything is smooth and completely mixed together. Place in the fridge to let cool and harden slightly while you prep the other ingredients.

- Spread the pecan halves across a baking sheet in an even layer and toast in the oven for 5-7 minutes until the pecans become fragrant and slightly browned. Remove the pecans from the oven and let cool.
- Add about an inch of water to a medium sauce pot and bring to a simmer. Add the chocolate to a heat proof bowl. Make sure the heat proof bowl is large enough that it can sit in the sauce pot without actually sitting the pot or touching the bottom of the pot. Stir the chocolate as it softens over the simmering water. When there are only a few chocolate chunks left unmelted, remove the bowl from the heat. Keep stirring until the chocolate is fully melted. Set aside.

- Line a couple of baking sheets with parchment paper and arrange the pecan halves into star shaped clusters of five. You can also just drop the pecans into small clusters without arranging them. They won't look like turtles, but it will be faster and just as delicious in the end.
- Remove the caramel mixture from the fridge. If the caramel has solidified stir until it becomes easier to work with - the consistency should be like honey or brown rice syrup.
- Use a small spoon to drop mounds over the pecan clusters. Do this until all of the pecan clusters are covered.
- Use another small spoon to cover each pecan caramel cluster with the melted dark chocolate chocolate. Once every cluster is covered, place in the refrigerator to let harden for 20 minutes and enjoy.

Nutrition Info

Calories: 179 Saturated Fat: 3g Sodium: 29mg Carbohydrates: 10g Fiber: 2g Sugar: 7g Protein: 2g

68 Vegan Cornbread Muffins with Aquafaba

Prep Time 10 minutes
Cook Time 20 minutes
Total Time 30 minutes
Servings: 12

Ingredients

- 1 cup cornmeal, 120 grams
- 1 cup gluten free all-purpose flour, 140 grams
- 1 teaspoon baking powder
- 1/4 teaspoon salt
- 1/2 cup melted coconut oil, 105 grams
- 1/3 cup packed light brown sugar, 67g
- 3 tablespoons aquafaba, water from cans of chickpeas
- 1 cup dairy free milk, 240ml, at room temperature

Instructions

- Preheat the oven to 400°F/205°C
- In a large mixing bowl whisk together the cornmeal, gluten free all purpose flour, baking powder, and salt. Set aside.
- In a medium sized mixing bowl add the aquafaba. Beat the aquafaba with an electric mixer on high for 3-4 minutes or until the aquafaba becomes white and glossy. Add the coconut oil and brown sugar and mix to combine.

- Pour the aquafaba and brown sugar mixture into dry ingredients. Add the milk and mix it all together until it's all fully combined.
- Spoon the batter into greased muffin tins to the top. Bake in the oven for 15-20 minutes or until a tooth pick inserted into the center comes out clean.
- Run a knife around the sides of the muffins to loosen them from the tray and remove from the tin to cool.

Nutrition Info

Calories: 189 Saturated Fat: 7g Sodium: 78mg Carbohydrates: 23g Fiber: 2g Sugar: 6g Protein: 2g

69 Mini Paleo Salmon Cakes & a Lemony Herb Aioli

Prep Time 15 minutes
Cook Time 30 minutes
Total Time 45 minutes
Servings: 10

Ingredients

- 2 1/4 cups | 12 oz. cooked salmon, flaked
- 1/4 cup mashed or pureed sweet potato or white potatoes, see notes
- 4 green onions, green parts only for low FODMAP, chopped
- 1 tablespoon fresh parsley, chopped
- 1 tablespoon dijon mustard

- 1 teaspoon lemon zest
- 1 tablespoon lemon juice
- 3 tablespoons capers, liquid drained
- 1 egg, beaten
- 3/4 teaspoon sea salt
- 1/2 teaspoon ground black pepper
- Lemon wedges for serving

Lemon Herb Aioli
- 1 egg yolk
- 1 tablespoon fresh lemon juice
- 1/2 teaspoon dijion mustard
- 1/2 cup garlic infused olive oil for low FODMAP or regular olive oil
- 1 large clove garlic, omit for low FODMAP
- 1 tablespoons fresh parsley, chopped
- 1 teaspoon fresh dill, chopped

Instructions
- Preheat the oven to 350°/180°C
- In a large mixing bowl, add all of the salmon cake ingredients. Mix everything together with a fork util combined. Form mini patties, about 3 inches in diameter and place on the baking tray. Bake for 25-30 minutes or until firm and browned on the sides. Make sure to flip the patties over in the oven halfway through cook time.

Lemon Herb Aioli
- While the salmon cakes are baking make the aioli. The easiest way to make this is with an immersion blender but you can also make this in a food processor, blender, or using an electric mixer.
- Place the egg yolk, 1/2 of the lemon juice, and mustard in a small bowl or blender/processor. Start whisking/blending everything together until the mixture thickens. Then gradually pour in the olive oil. It's important to add the oil

slowly because adding too much too soon will result in a runny or cuddled aioli. As the mixture thickens, add more oil until you have a thick, creamy mayo.

- Add the remaining lemon juice along with the garlic, parsley, and dill and mix in by hand. Taste and season with salt if needed. Transfer the aioli to a small bowl and serve with the salmon cakes. Store left overs in an airtight container in the fridge for up to a week.

Nutrition Info

Calories: 61 Cholesterol: 35mg Sodium: 281mg Carbohydrates: 1g Protein: 7g

Conclusion

A healthy renal diet can help retain kidney function for longer. The main differences between any healthy diet and a renal diet, are the restrictions placed on protein and table salt intake. Restrictions on phosphorus, potassium and fluids may become necessary as symptoms and signs of accumulation become evident.

Following renal diet guidelines will help decrease the workload on damaged kidneys and slow down the loss of kidney function. The renal diet guidelines are intended to help keep kidney sufferers healthy and functional by eating to support and augment their treatment. It is very important to get specific advice from your doctor and dietitian at all times.

Part 2

Introduction

Overtime, chronic kidney disease has become a global issue. Every now and then we hear tragic stories of people that have chronic kidney disease. However, the big news here is that chronic kidney disease is not the end of the world. It can be managed and treated if discovered early. The best way to manage chronic kidney disease is to adopt a new way of eating. This kidney friendly way of eating is what we call the renal diet. With the renal diet, you can manage chronic kidney disease and avoid dialysis. Dialysis can be stressful and costly.

This book features awesome low sodium and low potassium recipes that are good for people who have chronic kidney disease. This book also contains important pieces of information about the kidneys, chronic kidney disease and renal diet.

Chapter 1: the kidney

Since this book is all about kidney health, let's start my discussing the kidney and its importance to our body. The kidneys are two bean shaped fist-sized organs that can be found at the back of our abdominal cavity, just below the rib cage, on both sides of the spine. Our kidneys are so close to our back that it may be a bit difficult for a lay man to differentiate between back pain and kidney pain.

Physically, our kidneys are a bit small. Each kidney is about 4 to 5 inches long. But guess what! Their importance to the body system cannot be overemphasized. The kidneys perform important functions that are essential for the well being of the entire body. In fact, no human can survive if these functions are not executed. The kidneys are the body's filtration and waste management powerhouse. As such, if anyone suffers kidney failure, there is a need to find an alternative way to carry out the functions of the kidneys in the body if the person wants to survive. That brings us to the issue of dialysis, which shall be discussed later in this book. Those beans below your rib cage are not there for decoration!

So, if the kidneys are so important to our body system, what then is the job description of the kidneys in our body and why are the kidney functions indispensable to our body?

Functions of the kidneys

The kidneys filter the blood

At every point in time, the kidneys are busy filtering the blood in our body to get rid of waste and excess fluid in the body. On the average, your kidneys filters about 7.5 liters of blood per hour. Our kidneys house about a million filtering units that are medically referred to as "nephrons". Each of these nephrons is made up of glomerulus (a cluster of tiny blood vessels) and these tiny blood vessels are responsible for filtering blood in our body.

During the digestive process, your body absorbs the nutrients in the foods you eat. Afterwards, the absorbed nutrients are used to feed your cells and repair your cells. Absorbed nutrients are also converted to energy to power your brain. Once your body has utilized the amount of nutrients needed at a point in time, excess nutrients are released into the blood as waste products. Urea, salt and creatinine constitute a larger percentage of these waste products. The problem here is that waste products released into the blood can build up and become toxic overtime if not discarded. This is where the kidneys come in to rescue the body from the danger of allowing waste products to build up in the blood stream.

As the heart is pumping oxygen filled blood to all parts of the body, blood with wastes flows into our kidneys through the renal arteries. As the blood flows into our kidney, it is distributed into the nephrons, where it is filtered by a cluster of tiny blood vessels called glomerulus. The glomeruli have the capacity to filter out the waste in the blood. Each glomerulus is so tiny that only smaller molecules can pass through it. These smaller molecules constitute the waste products in our blood. As such, when our blood is filtered by the glomeruli, the smaller molecules are allowed to flow into the tubules as waste while larger molecules which include protein and red blood cells are retained. After filtration, filtered blood, containing protein and red blood cells is released back into our body system through the renal veins. The waste products will eventually be transported into the bladder through the ureters as urine.

This is how the kidney filters our blood everyday to avoid the buildup of toxic waste in the bloodstream. If your kidneys fail, waste products will start building up in your body. This can lead to a lot of crisis medically and eventually lead to death. I like to compare the importance of kidneys, as the ultimate blood filters, to the body to that of a fuel filter to a car engine. If car's fuel filter is bad, the engine will get clogged up with dirt and it may eventually stop working if the issue is not attended to. Likewise, if anyone suffers kidney failure, their blood will get clogged up with toxins and this may lead to a lot of negative health issues or death if not attended to immediately.

B. The kidneys regulate your body water/fluid

The kidneys play the most significant role in balancing the water content in our body. Our body's water content needs to be balanced as excess body fluid or insufficient body fluid can cause problems in our body system. This function of the kidneys can be described in two different situations.

On the one hand, when the water content in our body is excess, the kidneys perform a significant role in ensuring that excess water is removed from the blood and excreted to keep our body fluid balanced.

How is this done?

The excretion of excess water from our body takes a cause and effect format, one state stimulating the occurrence of other activities in the body. When we consume excess water, it will dilute our blood and increase the volume of blood in the body. Once the volume of blood increases, the hydrostatic pressure of our blood will rise above normal. Consequently, our kidneys will respond to this by increasing ultrafiltration – the filtration of blood by the glomeruli. With increased ultrafiltration, the rate at which the glomeruli filter the blood will increase, thereby enhancing the prompt removal of excess water from the blood.

During the filtration process, excess water will be transported to the bladder through the ureters to form urine. In cases like this, the urine content is usually diluted and less yellowish. So, whenever you go into the toilet to pass out a lot of diluted urine content, it means that your kidneys have worked hard to get rid of excess fluid from your blood.

On the other hand, the kidneys are also saddled with the responsibility of increasing our body's fluid content when the body is dehydrated. This is normally achieved through the process of reabsorption. The kidneys in conjunction with the hypothalamus perform a significant role in balancing body fluid during dehydration. Our body loses water every day through urine, sweat, breathing and even evaporation of water from the skin, especially during sunny days. Thus, it is important for us to drink enough water every day to replenish lost water content. But if you do not drink enough water at a point in time, you may be dehydrated.

During dehydration, your blood plasma will become thicker because it contains less water content. Once this happens, it will trigger some activities in your body system. These activities will start from the hypothalamus - a small region of our brain located at the base of the brain, near the pituitary gland. The hypothalamus, through the posterior pituitary gland, will release a hormone called the antidiuretic hormone (ADH) into the body system. This hormone will then send a signal to the kidney to reabsorb water from urine in order to dilute blood plasma. In response to this signal, the nephron in the kidney will start reabsorbing water and solute from the waste in the tubules. Reabsorbed water will then be released into the blood to dilute the blood plasma. This process is responsible for the formation of concentrated yellowish urine.

The foregoing processes explain how the kidney regulates our body fluid content. I guess you now see one more reason why the kidneys are so important to our body system.

C. The kidneys aid the creation of red blood cells in our body

The kidneys also play a vital role in preventing anemia by aiding the production of red blood cells in our body. Healthy kidneys are responsible for the production of a hormone called erythropoietin (EPO). EPO is essential for the production of red blood cells in our body. The function of the red blood cells is to circulate oxygen to body organs and tissues so that they can function properly. This means that a reduction in the amount of red blood cells in our body will result in to a reduction in the supply of oxygen in our body, thereby reducing the effectiveness of body organs and tissues in our body. Anytime the kidney senses a reduction in body oxygen, it will produce erythropoietin (EPO). EPO will then stimulate our bone marrows to produce more red blood cells in other to increase body oxygen circulation and regulate the function of body organs and tissue. The parts of our kidney that produce EPO are called the juxtaglomerular cells – cells that are close to the glomerulus.

D. The kidneys regulate blood pressure

Apart from the fact that the kidneys regulate blood pressure by getting rid of excess blood fluid, the kidneys also contribute to the regulation of blood pressure by regulating blood potassium level, regulating blood sodium level and also producing renin – a hormone which is essential for regulating blood pressure.

Sodium and potassium are two electrolytes that have a major effect on our blood pressure level. Sodium is responsible for increasing blood pressure and potassium is responsible for reducing blood pressure. If blood sodium is too low or the blood potassium is too high, it will lead to low blood pressure. Likewise, if blood sodium is too high or blood potassium is too low, blood pressure will rise. It is the job of our kidneys to keep our blood sodium level and potassium level balanced in order to regulate blood pressure.

Whenever the kidneys sense an abnormal reduction in blood pressure, the kidneys will produce and release renin into the blood stream. Renin will then convert angiotensinogen (a precursor protein that is primarily produced and released by the liver) into angiotensin 1. Subsequently, angiotensin 1 will be converted to angiotensin 2 in the lungs by an enzyme called Angiotensin-Converting Enzyme (ACE). Once angiotensin 2 is formed it will constrict the blood vessels in our body, thereby causing blood pressure to increase.

Angiotensins 2 will also stimulate the production of another hormone called aldostrone in the adrenal gland. When aldostrone is released, it will stimulate the renal tubules to increase the reabsorption of sodium and water into the blood stream and increase the excretion of potassium from the blood. This action will also increase blood pressure.

E. The kidneys promote bone health

Our kidneys are essential for maintaining healthy bones because they actively regulate the level of calcium and phosphorus in our body.

The kidneys aid bone health by activating vitamin D. The foods will consume contain an inactive form of vitamin D, which is usually activated by the kidney. When the kidney activates vitamin D, it is converted into calcitriol which facilitates the absorption of calcium by our intestine and indirectly improve bone health. Without calcitriol, our intestine cannot absorb calcium and the inability of the intestine to absorb calcium will lead to bone weakness. Calcitriol helps the kidneys to maintain blood calcium and improve bone health.

The kidneys also aid bone health by getting rid of excess phosphorous in our body. Although our body needs phosphorous to form and repair our bones and teeth, excess blood phosphorous can extract calcium from our bones and cause bone weakness. To avoid this, the kidneys are needed to filter out excess blood phosphorus into the urinary tubules during filtration.

Chronic Kidney Disease

Having discussed the functions and importance of the kidneys, let us talk about Chronic Kidney Disease (CKD), causes of chronic kidney diseases and the symptoms of chronic kidney disease. Kidney disease is a condition where the kidneys can no longer perform their functions effectively. Kidney disease is not spontaneous; it happens gradually and in stages. In fact, people with kidney disease may not notice that they have kidney disease until kidney functions have reduced immensely. Kidney disease is chronic; that is, it cannot be cured. However, it can be treated or managed, particularly in the early stages of the disease. If kidney disease is not treated immediately, it will lead to kidney failure. And when that happens, the only way the patient can survive is through dialysis or kidney transplant. We shall talk about dialysis and kidney transplant in this book later. And remember, the purpose of this book is to help chronic kidney disease patients to avoid dialysis/ kidney transplant. Now, let us look into the causes of Chronic Kidney Disease (CKD).

Causes of Chronic Kidney Disease (CKD)
A. Diabetes

Uncontrolled diabetes has been reported to be the leading cause of kidney disease. A lot of medical studies have proved that diabetes patients are at high risk of chronic kidney disease (CKD). Diabetes is another chronic disease that causes an abnormal increase in blood sugar. Abnormal increase in blood sugar will increase the level of waste product in our blood, thereby giving the kidney more work to do. If this continues uncontrolled over time, the glomerulus will worn out and start to leak as a result of constant excess work. This will result to a decrease in the effectiveness of the kidney as the glomerulus would have expanded and they would not be able to retain blood proteins anymore. Thus, protein contents that should be retained in the blood will now be released into the tubules and excreted as urine. This is the reason for the presence of protein in the urine of chronic kidney disease (CKD) patients. It is advisable for diabetes patients to go for kidney disease test to be sure that their kidneys are healthy.

B. High blood pressure

High blood pressure ranks as the second leading cause of chronic kidney disease (CKD). Blood pressure is the force by which blood flows through our body. When blood pressure is high, it will start to strain the blood vessels in the body. If this condition continues uncontrolled over time, it will damage body blood vessels, including the ones in the kidney. Once the glomeruli (tiny blood vessels in the kidneys) are damaged, their blood filtration rate will start to decrease gradually until they are unable to filter blood again. The inability of the kidney to filter blood is called kidney failure- the last stage of chronic kidney diseases. If you have high blood pressure, you have to take necessary measures to regulate your blood pressure and also go for a kidney disease test to ensure that your kidneys are healthy. Chronic kidney disease is best treated and managed when it is discovered early.

C. Glomerulonephritis

This is another leading cause of kidney disease. Glomerulonephritis is a disease that affects our glomerulus. It causes an abnormal inflammation of the glomerulus, thereby reducing the effectiveness of the glomerulus. If this condition persists over time, it can lead to kidney failure. There are two types of glomerulonephritis: (i) acute glomerulonephritis and (ii) chronic glomerulonephrtis. Acute glomerulonephritis happens suddenly and it is usually triggered by the effect of other diseases such as strep throat infection, lupus, good pasture syndrome and polyarteritis. Chronic glomerulonephritis on the other hand is usually hereditary. The symptoms of glomerulonephritis include:

I.   Blood urine
II. Swelling in the ankles and face
III. Urinating less often
IV. Puffiness of the face, especially in the morning
V.   Foamy urine
VI. High blood pressure
VII. Nosebleeds
VIII.   Abdominal pain
IX. Urinating frequently at nighttime

It is highly important for you to visit your doctor for check up immediately if you notice any of these symptoms. Untreated glomerulonephritis will cause irreversible damage to your kidneys and can lead to kidney failure. It is advisable for people who have history of chronic glomerulonephritis in their family to go for check up periodically to ensure good kidney health.

D. Polycystic kidney disease (PKD)

Polycystic kidney disease, just like chronic glomerulonephritis, is genetic. People who have polycystic kidney disease (PKD) inherited it from one of their parents or both. Polycystic kidney disease causes a cluster of cysts (noncancerous fluid filled sac-like bumps that can develop in any part of the body) to develop in the kidney. Development of cyst in the kidneys will make the kidneys swell abnormally and reduce their effectiveness. If this condition is not managed properly, it can lead to kidney failure. Common symptoms of polycystic kidney disease include:

i.   Joint pain
ii.   Abdominal pain
iii. Fatigue
iv.   Nail abnormalities
v.   Kidney stones
vi.   Constant back pain
vii. Pain in the kidney area (your back and loin, just below the rib cage)
viii. Bruises
ix.   Blood in urine

E. Kidney stones

Kidney stones, also known as nephrolithiasis, can also cause chronic kidney disease (CKD) and lead to kidney failure if it is not treated on time. Kidney stones are crystal-like mineral formations that can develop in the kidneys, bladder, ureters as well as in the urethra. Kidney stones usually develop when your urine is too concentrated. Some of the concentrated minerals or waste products in the urine may start to stick together, forming kidney stones. Concentrated urine can be prompted by dehydration, inflammatory bowel disease, persistent consumption of excess salt, protein or glucose, renal tubular acidosis, obesity, chronic diarrhea, hyparathyrodism and some other medical conditions. Some types of kidney stone disease are also hereditary. Calcium formed kidney stones are the most common type of kidney stone. Kidney stones can also be formed by uric acid, cystine, xanthine and phosphate. The easiest way to prevent kidney stones is by drinking enough water every day. You should drink about 10 glasses of water or more every day. This will help to dilute your urine and prevent the formation of concentrated urine.

People with kidney stones are at higher risk of chronic kidney disease (CKD) Kidney stones, especially the ones that are not too big, can eventually be passed out as urine but some of them can get to obstruct some tracts in the kidney and trigger kidney disease. Common symptoms of kidney stones include:

I. Blood urine
II. Painful urination
III. Smelling urine
IV. Pain in the kidney area (your side and back, below your rib cage)
V. Nausea and vomiting
VI. Pain in the lower abdominal area
VII. Fever and chills

If you sense one or more of these symptoms, you should visit your doctor immediately for check up. People whose family has a history of kidney stone should also go for check up periodically to be sure that their kidneys are free from stones.

F. Kidney Trauma

This is when parts of our kidneys are damaged as a result of an external force. There are two types of kidney trauma: blunt kidney trauma and penetrating trauma. Blunt trauma is usually caused by, car accident, fall or assault while penetrating trauma results from gunshot or stabbing. Kidney trauma can trigger chronic kidney disease. In fact, kidney trauma, especially penetrating, trauma can lead to acute kidney failure if it is not treated immediately. The kidneys of patients who are victims of severe back injury, abdominal injury, rib fractures, car accident, gunshot, stabbing and assault should be examined immediately. Symptoms of kidney trauma include:

I. Hematura - blood in the urine
II. Skin bruising
III. Skin discoloration

IV. Low blood pressure
V. Pain in the kidney area (your back and sides, below the rib cage)
VI. Anemia

No form of kidney trauma is minor; kidney injury sustained during trauma can pave way for chronic kidney disease as well as acute kidney failure. If you are a victim of car accident, assault, gunshot or stabbing, visit a doctor immediately. Our kidneys happen to be one of those body organs that are very susceptible to injury during accidents.

G. Drugs and toxins

A number of chronic kidney disease cases stem from the adverse effects of some drugs on our renal system. More people are now fond of misusing drugs due to the increase in the production of different drugs and the easy accessibility to these drugs. Self medication has become the order of the day; people just go to the counter to buy drugs without prescription. This has lead to an increase in cases of chronic kidney disease because our kidneys are quite susceptible to the adverse effects of drug abuse. Our kidneys are at the receiving end here because they are saddled with the responsibility of removing the excess toxins released into the blood as a result of improper drug usage.

Such drugs include antibiotics; non steroidal anti inflammatory drugs (NSAID) such as ibuprofen and aspirin; laxatives; supplements; diuretics and aminoglycosides (AMG). I do not think we really need to give a long list of all these drugs. The bottom line here is that you should stay away from using drugs without prescription. And if you have been abusing the use of any of the listed drugs or other drugs, please visit your doctor to check if your kidneys have not been affected.

H. Smoking

Smokers are at high risk of chronic kidney disease (CKD) and kidney cancer. Smoking can affect the kidneys in a lot of ways, directly and indirectly. To start with, smoking can affect your kidney health indirectly because it can trigger high blood pressure, which is a leading cause of kidney disease. Smoking also tightens blood vessels in the body. This usually results into slow flow of blood and oxygen to the body organs, including the kidneys. The kidneys, just like all body organs, need blood and oxygen to function properly; thus, their effectiveness will reduce when they are not getting enough blood and oxygen. This can eventually trigger chronic kidney disease (CKD).

More so, nicotine, one of the components of a cigarette, can facilitate the progression of damage in kidney disease patients. As such, patients of chronic kidney disease as well as people with healthy kidneys should stay away from smoking. Abstaining from smoking can be a little bit difficult because of the addictive effect of nicotine, but if you really want your kidneys to be healthy or you want to avoid dialysis, you need to stop smoking now.

Common symptoms of Chronic Kidney Disease

One funny thing about chronic kidney disease is that people who have the disease do not normally sense the symptoms during the early stage of the disease. Most people get to sense the symptoms when the effectiveness of the kidneys has decreased greatly. And even when some of the symptoms are noticed, some people do not recognize these symptoms or pay attention to them. In fact, some people may not know that they have chronic kidney disease (CKD) until their kidney fails. So, do not be surprised when you are told that your neighbor who played table tennis with you a day before collapsed on the next day while cooking as a result of critical kidney condition. Let us quickly look into some of the symptoms of chronic kidney disease (CKD).

A. Anemia induced fatigue

Anemia is a negative health condition that has to do with the insufficiency of red blood cells in the body. The red blood cells transport blood and oxygen to all organs and tissues of the body. Body organs need the oxygen circulated by red blood cells to function effectively. As hinted earlier, a kidney secreted hormone, Erithropoetin (EPO), is essential in the production of more red blood cells in the body. When you have chronic kidney disease (CKD) your kidneys may stop producing enough EPO. This will in turn affect the availability of enough red blood cells in the body. In this light, your body organs, including the brain, will not be getting enough oxygen. This will cause weakness in your body organs and lid to fatigue.

B. Memory loss or inability to concentrate

This symptom comes with anemia. It is as a result of insufficient supply of oxygen to the brain.

C. Bone weakness

When the kidneys are damaged, they may not be able maintain the balance of calcium and phosphorus in the body. Thus, your bones will start getting weak.

On the one hand, your blood calcium level will decrease. Calcitrol, the active form of vitamin D which is usually activated by the kidney, is responsible for the absorption of calcium by the intestines. When your kidneys are not at their best, there may be a reduction in the production of calcitrol. This will reduce the absorption of calcium from foods and decrease blood calcium level. Thus, your bones may start to weaken as your bones need enough calcium to stay healthy.

On the other hand, chronic kidney disease can lead to the availability of too much phosphorus in the blood. Unhealthy kidneys will not be able to filter out excess phosphorus from the blood. Excess phosphorus is quite inimical to your bone health. Although phosphorus is essential for bone health, excess phosphorus will extract calcium from the bones and cause bone weakness.

D. Foamy urine

When the glomerulus in your kidneys are no longer effective, protein contents that should be retained in the blood will be escaping into the tubules to form urine. The presence of protein in your urine will cause your urine to foam. Foamy urine is a common symptom of chronic disease. Unfortunately, most people do not pay attention to their urine when they urinate.

E. Swelling legs, feet and ankles / puffy eyes

Chronic Kidney disease causes toxins and excess mineral to start building up in the blood as the kidneys will be unable to get rid of these waste products. Over time, these toxins and excess mineral will start lodging in your legs, feet, ankle, joints and face. If you notice any abnormal swelling in one or more of these areas, visit your doctor immediately. Chronic kidney disease (CKD) is best managed when it is discovered early.

F. Constant back pain

This is one symptom of chronic kidney disease (CKD) that people don't take seriously. I guess we all see back pain as a normal thing. Chronic kidney disease can cause constant pain in your lower back area, below the rib cage. If you notice constant pain in your groin or lower back area, you should visit your doctor for check up. Pain relief drugs may not help things here.

G. High blood pressure

Unhealthy kidneys are unable to regulate blood fluid level. This allows minerals like sodium to build up in the body. The presence of excess fluid and sodium in the blood stream will increase your blood pressure level. Another bad news here is that increased blood pressure can cause more damage to the kidneys. Remember, high blood pressure is the second leading cause of kidney disease. As such, it is very important for high blood patients to take kidney disease tests periodically.

H. Nausea and vomiting

The presence of excessive fluid in the blood stream as a result of chronic kidney disease can make you nauseate and vomit. Though nauseating and vomiting are symptoms of different health conditions, it is advisable to always visit a doctor to know the cause of it. Don't just go to the chemist to get drugs; visit a doctor to know the true cause of the nausea and vomiting.

I.   Dry and Itchy skin

The buildup of excessive fluid, especially phosphorus, in the blood can cause your skin to itch. Excessive build up of urea on the blood can also cause your skin to be dry. Itchy skin also comes with anemia, which is one of the complications of chronic kidney disease. Cases of dry itchy skin should be given prompt medical attention.

J.   Loss of appetite and abnormal changes in food taste

Excessive blood fluid can also affect your taste bud. Foods will start tasting metallic to you and you may start losing appetite.

K. Shortness of breath

When excess fluid starts building up in your blood as a result of unhealthy kidneys, they will start lodging in your body organs including the lungs. The presence of excess fluid in the lungs can cause shortness of breath. Cases of shortness of breath should be given prompt attention medically. Put yourself together and go for a checkup.

115

L. Bad breath

People with chronic kidney disease can have bad breath as a result of the deposit of excess fluid and electrolytes in the blood and body organs.

M. Feeling cold always

The buildup of excess fluid and minerals in the blood can pave way for hypothermia - a state where the body temperature drops abnormally. Kidney disease patient may also feel cold always as a result of limited red blood cells in their body.

N. Muscle cramp

Frequent muscle cramps, especially leg cramp, are also a symptom of chronic kidney disease (CKD). High blood pressure, a common symptom of chronic kidney disease (CKD), can stretch and narrow the blood vessels in legs. This may cause frequent leg cramps in people who have chronic kidney disease. Frequent muscle cramps can also be triggered by the presence of excess fluid and electrolytes in the blood. If you have been having frequent muscle cramps, especially leg cramps, visit a doctor for check up.

If you notice one or more of these highlighted symptoms of chronic kidney disease (CKD), do not hesitate to visit your doctor for proper check up.

Stages of Chronic Kidney Disease (CKD)

Chronic kidney disease (CKD) is not a sudden condition; it occurs in stages. Patients move from one stage of chronic kidney disease to the other as the effectiveness of the kidneys decreases over time until they get to the last stage. The last stage of chronic kidney disease is kidney failure. At this stage, patients need dialysis or kidney transplant to survive.

Stages of chronic kidney disease are identified according to a patient's estimated Glomerular Filtration Rate (GFR) - the rate at which the kidney filters toxins from the blood. GFR is considered the yardstick for measuring overall kidney functions.GFR is usually determined by examining the level of blood creatinine, a waste product that is produced during muscle metabolism, in conjunction with other factors such as age, sex, body size and race. . Let us highlight the stages of chronic kidney disease (CKD).

Stage 1

At stage one, the functions of the kidneys are still normal and patients may not notice any obvious symptoms. But protein can be noticed in patients' urine if tested. The estimated glomerular filtration rate (GFR) of the kidneys at stage one is 90 ml per minute or above. This is similar to GFR of a healthy kidney.

Stage 2

Stage two chronic kidney disease (CKD) characterizes a mild decrease in kidney functions. At this point, a little rise in the level of creatinine in the blood can be noticed if the patient is tested. The estimated glomerular filtration rate (GFR) of the kidney in stage two is around 60 to 89 ml per minute.

Stage 3

 Stage 3 is often referred to as the middle stage of chronic kidney disease (CKD). It is the most common category of chronic kidney disease. At stage 3 there is a moderate decrease in kidney functions and patients must have started to sense some complications of chronic kidney disease. These complications include anemia, high blood pressure, bone weakness and fatigue. The third stage of chronic kidney disease (CKD) occurs in two phases. The estimated glomerular filtration rate (GFR) for phase one stage 3 of CKD is around 45 to 59 ml per minutes while phase two features an estimated GFR of 30 to 44 ml per minute.

Stage 4

At stage four, the functions of the kidney will have decreased immensely and the patient will be faced with a lot of negative health conditions associated with chronic kidney disease (CKD). This stage is associated with severity. At this stage, doctors will already be planning for dialysis or kidney transplant. The estimated glomerular filtration rate (GFR) in stage four is around 15 to 29 ml per minute.

Stage 5

Stage five is the last stage of chronic kidney disease. This is the stage where the kidneys finally fail. The estimated glomerular filtration rate (GFR) is below 15 ml per minutes. The kidneys may still be able to function a bit but the level of the kidney functions at this stage will not be enough to keep the patient alive. At stage five the patient will need dialysis or kidney transplant to survive.

Chapter two

treatments for kidney failure (ckd)

There are two treatments for chronic kidney disease (CKD): dialysis and kidney transplant.

Dialysis

The main purpose of this book is to help chronic kidney disease patients to maintain the condition in order to avoid dialysis. Thus, it is important that we talk about dialysis. Dialysis, also known as kidney replacement therapy, is a process of getting rid of waste products, toxins, excess fluid and electrolytes from the blood of kidney failure patients. Dialysis gives hope to people whose kidneys have failed. There are two main types of dialysis: Hemodialysis and peritoneal dialysis.

A. Hemodialysis

Hemodialysis is a type of dialysis that is performed with the use of a dialysis machine. Blood will be passed into the machine via a tube connected to an "access" (we shall talk about "access" later under this subtopic). The machine will then filter the blood to get rid of excess fluid and waste product from the blood. There is a part of the dialysis machine called the dialyzer. The dialyzer acts a filter during hemodialysis. It is modeled after the glomeruli. The dialyzer ensures that toxins and waste products are filtered out of the blood while protein and red blood cells, which are too big to escape the filter, are retained. After filtration, clean blood containing protein and red blood cells will then be released into the blood via another tube. Patients usually undergo hemodialysis thrice in a week and each hemodialysis session can last up to four hours or more depending on the amount of waste in the blood and the capacity of the dialysis machine. Hemodialysis is the most preferred dialysis treatment to most kidney failure patients.

What is an access?

When chronic kidney disease (CKD) gets to the fourth stage in a patient, doctors will start preparing for dialysis or kidney transplant. If the chosen kidney failure treatment is hemodialysis, preparation includes creating a point in the body where blood can be accessed for hemodialysis. Access creation involves minor surgical operation. An access is created to ensure easy and fast flow of blood into the dialysis machine during hemodialysis. There are two main types of access: Fistula and graft

Fistula

To create a fistula, a doctor will join an artery and vein together in your arm (forearm or upper arm), under the skin to create a bigger blood vessel. A fistula is usually created few months to the commencement of dialysis so that the created blood vessel must have healed before then. During hemodialysis, two needles connected to two different tubes will be inserted into the fistula, one passing blood into the dialysis machine and the other releasing clean blood into the body.

Graft

A graft serves as a substitute to fistula in cases where the patient's blood vessels cannot be used to create a fistula. A graft is usually created by using a special soft tube to connect an artery and vein together, under the skin. A graft takes about four to six weeks to heal completely before they can be used for dialysis.

B. Peritoneal Dialysis

Peritoneal dialysis serves as an alternative to hemodialysis. Peritoneal dialysis is not entirely artificial; this type of dialysis makes use of the peritoneum as a dialyzer to filter the blood of the patient. The peritoneum is a serous membrane which lines and covers the abdominal cavity and the abdominal organs. This membrane acts as a natural filter through which waste is extracted from the blood during peritoneal dialysis.

How does peritoneal dialysis work?

Before the commencement of peritoneal dialysis, the patient needs to undergo a minor surgery in order to insert a permanent catheter into the patient's abdomen. The surgery will take a few weeks to heal before the catheter can be used for peritoneal dialysis.

During peritoneal dialysis, a cleansing fluid called dialysate will be released into a patient's abdomen through the catheter. Dialysate help to absorb waste products such as creatinine and urea from the blood flowing through the abdominal lining. The peritoneum allows waste to be released into the dialysate fluid while it retains useful blood contents such as red blood cells and protein. The dialysate will be allowed to stay in the abdomen for a specific time frame, about two hours or more. The specified time the dialysate spends in the patient's abdomen is refered to as the dwell time. After the dwell time, the dialysate which must have absorbed blood waste will be drain out of the stomach into a waste bag through the catheter. The bag to which the dialysate is drained is called the drainage bag. The drainage is to be removed and discarded after each dialysis. Peritoneal dialysis is quite simple to perform; it is usually done by the patients and it can be performed at work, at home or while traveling.

There are two types of peritoneal dialysis:

I. Continual Ambulatory Peritoneal Dialysis (CAPD)
II. Continuous Circling Peritoneal Dialysis (CCPD)

I. Continuous Ambulatory Peritoneal Dialysis (CAPD)

This form of peritoneal dialysis is usually performed manually, without the aid of any machine. The patient will first have to fill his or her abdomen with a bag of dialysate solution and later drain out the solution after the dwell time. The filling and draining system in continuous ambulatory peritoneal dialysis relies on gravity. The patient has to repeat the process three to four times daily with a new drainage bag and a new dialysate bag. The process of filling and draining dialysate solution from the abdomen in peritoneal dialysis is called exchange.

II. Continuous Circling Peritoneal Dialysis (CCPD)

This form of peritoneal dialysis is usually performed while the patient is sleeping with the aid of a machine known as the cycler. CCPD is also known as Automatic Peritoneal Dialysis (APD). All the patient has to do is to connect the cycler to the catheter before going to bed at night. While the patient is sleeping, the cycler will perform about 3 to 5 exchanges automatically. At each exchange, the cycle will fill the abdomen with dialysate and wait for the dwell time before draining the solution into a sterile bag. The sterile bag will be discarded by the patient in the morning. CCPD requires the patient to be connected to the cycler for about 10 to 12 hours every night. It means if you are the type that doesn't stay long in bed; you may have to adjust your sleeping habit to facilitate effective CCPD.

After the night's dialysis, the patient may need to carry out one manual exchange whose dwell time lasts the whole day. That is, you will allow the dialysate to remain in yourabdomen while you are out, doing your things during the day.

Kidney Transplant

Kidney transplant is another treatment for kidney failure. Kidney transplantation is a surgical operation performed to place a healthy kidney, removed from a donor, into a kidney failure patient. One amazing thing is that our body can function well with just one kidney. So, when a person's kidneys fail, another person can offer to donate one of their healthy kidneys to the kidney failure patient. After the kidney transplant, the patient and the donor can now live a healthy life with one healthy kidney each. In some cases, the donor may be deceased; healthy kidneys can be removed from someone who just died to replace that of a kidney failure patient. Thus, we have two categories of kidney transplantation: living-donor kidney transplantation and deceased donor kidney transplantation. Living donors are usually close relatives of the patient. To receive a healthy kidney from a deceased donor, you have to be on a national waiting list. The procedures for benefiting from deceased donor transplantation may vary across countries.

Chapter three

renal diet

Chronic kidney disease (CKD) cannot be cured as damages to parts of our kidneys are usually irreversible. However, the good news is that you can slow down the progression of the disease into critical stages by embracing a new lifestyle and way of eating. The kind of foods we eat indubitably has a great effect on the health of our body organs, including the kidneys. As a chronic kidney disease patient, the best thing to do is to switch to a kidney friendly diet. This kind of diet is popular known as the renal diet.

Although chronic kidney disease cannot be cured, the renal diet can help chronic kidney disease (CKD) patients to retain kidney functions and delay kidney failure for years. The major effect of the renal diet on our kidneys is that it reduces the workload of the kidney, thereby making them to last longer.

How is this achieved?

A proper renal diet is geared towards reducing the amount of sodium, phosphorus, potassium, protein and fluid consumed by a chronic kidney disease (CKD) patient. When this is achieved, the level of waste released into the blood after the body has extracted the useful materials in the food we eat will reduce. Consequently, the kidney will be relieved as they now have fewer waste products to filter. It would not cost the glomerulus much stress to filter the blood when the level of waste in the blood is low. Now, let us talk about how and why a chronic kidney disease (CKD) patient should regulate their intake of sodium, potassium, protein and phosphorus.

124

Sodium

Sodium is one of the essential electrolytes needed by our body. Sodium helps in regulating our blood pressure, balancing the level of water in our cells, facilitating proper muscle and nerves function and regulating the acid-base level of the blood.

Healthy kidneys get rid of excess sodium in our blood. However, damaged kidneys will not be to excrete excess blood sodium. This will result in the buildup of sodium in the blood. The consumption of excess sodium can negatively affect the kidneys of a chronic kidney disease patient in two ways. First, it will increase the workload of the damaged kidneys, thus causing more damages. Secondly, excess sodium will start to build up in the blood as a result of the kidneys inability to get rid of it. The buildup of excess sodium in the blood will lead to high blood pressure, a condition that can accelerate the progression of chronic kidney disease into critical stages and cause kidney failure.

As such, you have to watch the amount of sodium you consume per day. Try to limit your sodium consumption to 140 – 150 milligrams per serving for snacks and 400 – 500 mg per serving for meals. Generally, chronic kidney disease (CKD) patients are advised to keep their daily intake of sodium between 1500 to 2000 milligrams. However, you may need to consult a kidney dietitian to be sure of the right amount of sodium you are allowed to consume per day, depending on the condition of your kidneys and other variables.

How to control your sodium intake

1. Stay away from food containing high sodium:

When we talk about sodium consumption, some people think it's all about table salt, sea salt or other forms of salt. The fact is that some of the foods you eat are high in sodium even before you season them with salt. In fact, about 75% of the sodium we consume comes from the foods we eat, without added salt. Below is a list of foods containing high sodium:

Processed meats and fish

Smoked, canned, salted, picked or cure meats such as ham, bacon, pepperoni, regular canned salmon and tuna, sausage, wieners, deli meats, corn beef, salami, cold cuts, pepperoni, flakes of chicken, flakes of turkey, flakes of ham, potted meat, salted dried fish, salted smoked fish, salted fish, hot dogs, kosher meats, devilled ham, luncheon meat and so on.

Salt and salt seasonings

Salted mixed spices, seasoned pepper, lemon pepper, garlic salt, pink salt, seasoning salt, table salt, kosher salt, sea salt, bouillon cubes, flavor enhancers, onion salt, celery salt, lite salt, steak spice and so on.

Sauces

Soy sauce, barbeque sauce, teriyaki sauce, salted tomato sauce, tartar sauce, Worcestershire sauce, tobacco sauce, steak sauce, salted tomato sauce, Taco sauce, picante sauce, oyster sauce, chili sauce.

Condiments

Monosodium glutamate (MSG), salsa, meat tenderizers, ketchup, sauerkraut, salad dressing, olives, pickles and relish.

Canned foods

Salted canned soups, salted canned vegetables, canned juices, canned broths

Snacks

Salted snacks such as chips, pretzels, popcorn, cheezies, peanuts, salted crackers, pork rinds, salted nuts and so on.

Dairy and milk products

Butter milk, feta cheese, blue cheese, sweetened condensed milk, malted milk, processed cheese, Parmesan cheese, commercial milk drinks and so on.

Other high sodium foods include baking soda, baking powder, cheese bread, cookies, bacon fat, ovaltine, cream of tartar, corn syrup, salted butter, cheese bread, waffles, meat patties, instant potatoes, scalloped potato mix, salted margarine, salted mayonnaise, salted gravy and so on.

2. Pay attention to food nutritional fact labels

The list of both high sodium foods and low sodium foods is endless; you cannot know them all. So, when you go to the grocery store, always check nutritional fact labels to confirm if the food is low in sodium. Check for "sodium" on the food label and make sure the foods sodium content is equal to or less than 8% of your daily value. Foods containing more than 8% of your daily value of sodium per serving may not be good for your kidney health.

3. Go for fresh foods and homemade foods

Eating fresh foods reduces your sodium intake as fresh foods contain low sodium. In addition, go for homemade foods instead of packaged foods that may contain added sodium. When the food is homemade, you will be able to control the sodium content to suit your dietary needs. Eat fresh meat, beef, veal, pork, poultry, fish, vegetables, fruits, homemade soup, homemade broth, homemade sauce and so on.

4. Always pay attention to serving size

Most foods have a common serving size and their nutritional fact is usually estimated base on their specified serving size. Thus, it is not advisable for a chronic kidney disease patient to consume more than the given serving size of a food as this may cause excessive consumption of sodium even when the food has low sodium. For instance, if the serving size of a food is 100 grams and the sodium content per serving is 7% of your daily value, consuming 200 gram of that particular food per serving means you have consumed 14% of your daily value of sodium in one serving. Consuming 14% of your daily value of sodium intake at one serving is bad for your kidney health. There are common serving sizes; however, it is advisable that you go and consult a kidney dietitian to know the right serving size you are allowed to consume per meal for each food category according to the conditions of your kidneys.

5. Consume low sodium foods moderately

This is related to the issue of serving size. The fact that a food contains low sodium does not mean you should consume it excessively.

6. Use herb and spices to cook instead of salt or salt seasonings

Cultivate the habit of cooking without adding additional salt or salt seasonings. Rather, season your foods with herbs and spices moderately.

7. Go for unsalted foods

Check for phrases and words such as "no salt added" "unsalted" "sodium free" or "no sodium" on food packages. Food labeled with such words or phrases are usually safe to eat.

Potassium

Potassium is another essential electrolyte that performs important functions in our body. Potassium performs essential functions like supporting heart health, improving nerves and muscle functions, supporting bone health, balancing the fluid in and around our cells. When your kidneys are no longer functioning properly, they will be unable to get rid of excess potassium in the blood. This will result in an unhealthy buildup of potassium in your blood. An abnormal increase in blood potassium level is medically referred to as hyperkaliemia. Reducing your potassium consumption as a chronic disease is very important as hyperkaliemia can cause a lot of damages to your body. Consuming excess potassium can stress your unhealthy kidneys and make them worn out faster. In addition, excess build up of potassium in your blood stream as a result of the ineffectiveness of your kidneys can lead to low blood pressure- a negative health condition that can cause more damages to your kidneys. Generally, chronic kidney disease patients should not consume more than 1500 to 2300 milligrams of potassium per day. However, you may need to visit a kidney dietician to be sure of the right amount of potassium you should consume per day, depending on your kidney conditions and other variables.

How to regulate your potassium intake:

1. **Stay away from salt substitutes and seasonings that contain potassium**

Most salt substitutes and some seasonings contain potassium. Seasoning your food with salt substitutes or seasonings while cooking can result in excess potassium intake. Moreover, you should stay away from packages foods that contain salt substitute and potassium seasonings.

2. **Limit the consumption of high potassium foods**

All the foods we eat contain potassium; however, the potassium level of foods varies. Some foods are considered low in potassium while some are considered high in potassium. Foods that contain more than 200 mg of potassium per serving are considered high in potassium. As a chronic kidney disease patient, you have to limit your intake of high potassium foods and eat more low potassium foods. The list of high potassium foods include:

Fruits

Avocado, banana, medjool date, dried fruits, orange and orange juice, raisins, apricot, prunes and prune juice, pomegranate and pomegranate juice, sultanas, pumpkin, papaya, mango, nectarines, kiwi, honeydew melon, cantaloupe, fresh peaches, fresh pears, figs and melons.

Vegetables

Tomato, mushrooms, spinach, beetroot, dried beans, black kidney beans, pinto red beans, white beans, refried beans, chard, mustard, kale, spinach, turnip, collard, mustard, parsnips, yams, zucchini, winter squash, potatoes, artichokes, rutabagas, fried onions, broccoli, Brussels sprouts, kohlrabi, lentil and vegetable juice.

Nuts

Nuts are generally high in sodium.

Others

Processed meats, chocolate, puddings, yogurts, salt substitutes, peanut butter, nut butters, milk drinks, milk shakes, lentils, milk (evaporated milk, malted milk, soy milk, buttermilk), miso, seeds, tofu, creamed soups, ice cream, French fries, coconut, bran products, molasses, split peas , potato waffles, Hash browns and potato chips.

3. Eat more of low potassium foods

Your daily meals should feature more of low potassium foods. Such low potassium foods include:

Fruits

Apples, strawberry and strawberry nectar, pineapple, pineapple juice, apple sauce, apple juice, lime, raspberries, cranberry, cranberry juice, grape, grape juice, blueberries, blackberries, watermelon, tangerine, plums, mandarin oranges and fruit cocktail.

Vegetables

Carrots, onion, peas (green), alfalfa sprouts, eggplant, green beans, wax beans, lettuce, raw white mushrooms, peppers, cauliflower, cabbage, asparagus, celery, corn, radish, watercress, water chestnuts, cucumber, yellow squash, summer squash, okra, parsley, lemon and crookneck squash.

Other

Tortillas, rice, pasta, noodles, breads (excluding whole grain bread), alfafa seeds, regular oatmeal

4. Eat fresh and homemade food

Cooking at home and eating fresh foods gives you the opportunity to control your potassium intake. Packaged and processed foods may contain excess potassium.

5. Check food nutritional labels

Check nutritional labels on food packages to know their potassium content. Go for foods that contain less than 200 milligrams of potassium per serving. Foods containing more than 200 milligrams of potassium per serving may not be good for your kidney health.

6. Pay attention to serving size

Portion control is very important when following a renal diet. Do not consume more than one serving size of a food in one meal to avoid excess potassium intake. It is also advisable to visit a kidney dietician to know your perfect serving size for each food category, depending on your kidney condition and your body potassium level.

Phosphorous

Phosphorous is found in all foods and it is essential for our bones and muscle health. The kidneys are saddled with the responsibility of getting rid of excess phosphorous in our blood. Thus, when your kidneys are not healthy, excess phosphorous will start building up in your blood. Excess phosphorus will start extracting calcium from your bones, thereby causing severe bone weakness. To avoid this, you need to limit your phosphorous consumption if you have chronic kidney disease (CKD). Generally, chronic kidney disease patients should limit their phosphorous to 800 to 1000 milligrams per day. You should visit a kidney dietician to be sure of the right amount of potassium you are allowed to consume daily depending on the condition of your kidneys and other variables.

How to regulate your phosphorus consumption

1. Limit the consumption of foods that contain high phosphorous

All the foods we eat contain phosphorous; however, the amount of phosphorous content in food varies. Some foods contain high phosphorous content and some feature medium to low phosphorous. Foods containing less than 150 milligrams of phosphorous per serving have low phosphorous content, those containing 151 milligrams to 200 milligrams per serving are categorized under medium phosphorous foods and foods containing more than 200 milligrams per serving are considered to be high phosphorous foods. Chronic kidney disease patients should limit their consumption of high phosphorous foods. The list of high phosphorous foods includes:

Dairy and milk products

Goat cheese, part skim ricotta cheese, Romano cheese, parmesan cheese, buttermilk, chocolate milk, 1% milk, whole milk, low fat yogurt, skin yogurt, pudding, eggnog, soy milk, cream soup, custard, milk casseroles, condensed milk, evaporate milk, milk shake, non dairy creamers, processed cheese and non fat milk

Meat and protein foods

Pork, beef, tofu, beef liver, chicken liver, veal, lamb, organ meat, fish roe, processed meats, soy beans, beans, lentils, chickpeas, quinoa, amaranth and beefalo

Seafood

Fried calamari, oyster, sardine, blue mussels, crab clams, canned salmon, sole, swordfish, white tuna, light tuna, halibut, flounder, scallops and clam chowder

Beverages

Colas, beer, bottled ice tea, bottled fruit, punch and ale

Nuts and seeds

Almonds, peanuts, pine nuts, Brazil nuts, pecans, walnuts, pistachios, sunflower seeds, pumpkin seeds, chia seeds and cashews.

Others

Bran cereal, corn bread, wheat bread, whole grain breads, wheat flour and whole grain flour

2. Check ingredient labels on package foods

Take your time to check out for phosphorous or for words containing the morpheme "phos' on ingredient labels. Once you see phosphorous or any word containing "phos" on a food's ingredient labels, it means that the food contains added phosphorous. Please do your kidneys a favor by avoiding such packaged foods.

3. Consume high protein foods moderately

Protein rich foods naturally contain phosphorous. Foods that are high in protein usually contain high phosphorous content. Thus, high protein foods such as meat, dairy products, fish, poultry, nuts and beans should be consumed in smaller portions.

4. Use phosphate binders

Phosphate binders help to regulate the absorption of phosphorous in the foods we eat during digestion. Thus, taking phosphate binders at meal time can be used to control phosphorous consumption in CKD patients. However, you should consult a doctor or kidney dietician before using phosphate binders.

5. Check food nutritional fact labels

Check the nutritional fact labels on packaged foods. Select foods that contain less than 10% of your daily value of phosphorous intake. This may not be relevant in all cases as most food nutritional fact labels do not include phosphorous, even though the food contains phosphorous.

6. Pay attention to serving size

Do not consume more than one serving size of a food in a single meal. Eating more than one serving size of a low phosphorous food at a single meal can make a low phosphorous food become a high phosphorous food. Most foods have a common serving size; however, you may need to consult a dietician to know your perfect serving size for each food group.

7. Eat homemade and fresh foods

Cooking at home and eating fresh foods keeps you in control of your phosphorous consumption. You will be able to choose which foods to include in your meal, avoid phosphorous addictives and pay attention to serving size. Eating too much of packaged foods may not be good for kidneys.

Protein

Chronic kidney patients (CKD) also need to regulate their protein consumption. Protein is an essential macronutrient; it is need by our body to build muscles, fight infections, build tissues and heal wounds. People with healthy kidneys can eat high protein meals because their kidneys are active enough to excrete protein waste. However, CKD patients are advised to limit their protein intake as high protein intake can increase waste products in the blood and stress the kidneys. Limiting protein intake can be a bit tricky as insufficient intake of protein can also trigger some negative health conditions. Our body protein needs is determined by factors such as body size, sex and age. To stay safe, you need to consult a doctor or a kidney dietician to know the right amount of protein you should consume per day.

Fluid

Chronic kidney disease patient will also need to limit their daily consumption of liquids/fluids. Unhealthy kidneys do not have the capacity to effectively excrete excess body fluids. Thus, excess fluid will start to build up in the blood. The buildup of excess fluid in the blood can cause high blood pressure — a negative health condition that can accelerate the loss of kidney functions. This can also result in edema (swollen arms, joint, ankles, feet and legs).

Chapter four

kidney friendly homemade kitchen staples and seasonings

Beef Stock

PREP TIME: 5 minutes

COOK TIME: 4 hours 30 minutes

SERVINGS: 8 cups

Ingredients:

- 2 tbsp olive oil
- 9 cups water
- 2 pound beef bones (all fat trimmed)
- 2 fresh parsley stems
- ½ tsp curry powder
- ½ tsp thyme
- 2 celery stalks (chopped)
- 2 carrots (boiled without salt, drained and chopped)
- 1 tsp black peppercorns
- 1 bay leaf

Directions:

1. Preheat the oven to 440°F.
2. Arrange the beef bones into a deep baking pan and place the baking pan in the preheated oven.
3. Bake the beef bones for about 30 minutes.
4. Remove the baking pan from the oven. Add 1 tbsp olive oil and toss.
5. Add the carrot and celery.
6. Return the baking pan to the oven and bake the beef bones for another 30 minutes.
7. After the baking cycle, remove the baking pan from the oven and pour the roasted beef bones and veggies into saucepan.
8. Pour in the water and stir the parsley, black peppercorn, curry and thyme.
9. Add bay leave and bring the liquid to a boil over medium to high heat. Reduce the heat low and simmer the broth for 3 hours, covered. Check the broth at interval to skim off any foam or dirt that rises to the surface of the broth.
10. Remove the sauce pan from heat and leave the broth to cool for about 25 minutes.
11. Discard the bay leaf and strain the broth into a clean bowl with a fine mesh strainer.
12. Pour broth into containers and store in a refrigerator for up to six days. Always skim off excess fat from the surface of the broth before using.

Nutrition Facts

Servings: 8

Amount per serving

Calories	**195**

% Daily Value*

Total Fat 8.9g	**11%**
Saturated Fat 2.5g	**13%**
Cholesterol 76mg	**25%**
Sodium 76mg	**3%**
Total Carbohydrate 1.6g	**1%**
Dietary Fiber 0.7g	**2%**
Total Sugars 0.5g	
Protein 26.1g	
Vitamin D 0mcg	0%
Calcium 21mg	2%
Iron 16mg	91%
Potassium 60mg	

Relish

PREP TIME: 20 minutes

SERVINGS: 36 (1 tbsp per serving)

Ingredients:

- 1 cup chopped cucumber
- ¼ tsp cinnamon
- 1/8 tsp cayenne pepper
- 1 tsp celery seed
- 1/8 tsp allspice
- 1large onion (chopped)

- 2 cups chopped celery
- ½ cup sugar
- ¼ tsp ground mustard
- 1 small green pepper (chopped)
- 4 tbsp fresh chopped cilantro

Directions:

1. In a large mixing bowl, combine the cucumber, green pepper, cilantro, onion and celery.
2. Add the sugar, cinnamon, allspice, cayenne and mustard. Toss until the ingredients are well combined.
3. Cover the mixing bowl and place it in a mixing bowl. Chill for about 8 hours.

Nutrition Facts

Serving size: 1 tablespoon

Servings: 36

Amount per serving

Calories	**14**

% Daily Value*

Total Fat 0g	**0%**
Saturated Fat 0g	**0%**
Cholesterol 0mg	**0%**
Sodium 5mg	**0%**
Total Carbohydrate 3.6g	**1%**
Dietary Fiber 0.3g	**1%**
Total Sugars 3.1g	
Protein 0.1g	
Vitamin D 0mcg	0%
Calcium 5mg	0%
Iron 0mg	0%
Potassium 30mg	

Vegetable Stock

PREP TIME: 5 minutes

COOK TIME: 2 hours

SERVINGS: 6 cups

Ingredients:

- 7 cups of water

- 1 tsp black peppercorns
- 2 carrots (peeled and sliced)
- 1 onion (chopped)
- 4 garlic cloves (cloves)
- 4 celery stalks (chopped)
- 2 bay leaves
- 3 sprigs thyme
- 3 parsley sprigs

Directions:

1. Combine the water, parsley, garlic, onion, celery, bay leaves, peppercorns, carrots and thyme in a large sauce pan over medium to high heat.
2. Bring the mixture to a boil; cover the sauce pan; reduce the heat to medium-low and simmer the broth for about 2 hours, checking occasionally to skim off any fat that rises to the surface of the broth.
3. Remove the sauce pan from heat and discard the bay leaves.
4. Strain the vegetable broth into a clean bowl with a fine mesh strainer.
5. Pour the broth into jars and let it cool completely before sealing the jars.
6. Store the vegetable stock in the refrigerator for up to 5 days.

Nutrition Facts

Servings: 6

Amount per serving

Calories	**24**

% Daily Value*

Total Fat 0.1g	**0%**
Saturated Fat 0g	**0%**
Cholesterol 0mg	**0%**
Sodium 33mg	**1%**
Total Carbohydrate 5.4g	**2%**
Dietary Fiber 1.5g	**5%**
Total Sugars 2g	
Protein 0.7g	
Vitamin D 0mcg	0%
Calcium 41mg	3%
Iron 1mg	6%
Potassium 144mg	

Chicken Stock

PREP TIME: 5 minutes

COOK TIME: 2 hours

SERVINGS: 6 cups

Ingredients:

- 7 cups of water
- 2 pounds whole chicken (raw) cut into small bite sizes
- 1 bay leaf

- 1 black peppercorns
- 1 carrot (sliced)
- 1 onion (chopped)
- 4 celery stalks (chopped)
- 5 fresh thyme sprigs
- 3 fresh parsley stems

Directions:

1. Combine the chicken meat, thyme, celery, parsley, peppercorns, onion, carrot, bay leaf and water in a large sauce pan over medium to high heat.
2. Bring the mixture to a boil; reduce the heat to low and simmer the stock for about 2 hour, covered. Check the stock occasionally to skim off any foam or dirt on the surface of the stock.
3. Remove the sauce pan from heat and discard the bay leaf.
4. Strain the chicken stock into a clean bowl with a fine mesh strainer.
5. Pour the chicken stock into jars and let it cool completely before sealing the jars.
6. Store the chicken stock in a refrigerator for up to 7 days.

Nutrition Facts

Servings: 6

Amount per serving

Calories	**190**

% Daily Value*

Total Fat 11.5g	**15%**
Saturated Fat 3.4g	**17%**
Cholesterol 67mg	**22%**
Sodium 81mg	**4%**
Total Carbohydrate 3.5g	**1%**
Dietary Fiber 1.1g	**4%**
Total Sugars 1.5g	
Protein 14.6g	
Vitamin D 0mcg	0%
Calcium 42mg	3%
Iron 1mg	8%
Potassium 121mg	

Barbeque Sauce

PREP TIME: 5 minutes

COOK TIME: 5minutes

SERVINGS: 8 (2 tbsp per serving)

Ingredients:

- 5 tbsp + 1 tsp canola oil
- ¼ tsp onion powder
- 1 tbsp brown sugar

- ¼ cup vinegar
- 1 tbsp paprika
- ½ cup unsalted tomato juice
- 1 clove garlic (crushed)
- 1/3 cup water
- 1 tsp pepper

Directions:

1. Combine all the ingredients in a sauce pan.
2. Bring the mixture to a boil, reduce the heat and simmer the sauce for 20 minutes.
3. Pour leftover into a tightly sealed container and store in a refrigerator.

Nutrition Facts

Servings: 8

Amount per serving

Calories	95

% Daily Value*

Total Fat 9.4g	**12%**
Saturated Fat 0.7g	**4%**
Cholesterol 0mg	**0%**
Sodium 3mg	**0%**
Total Carbohydrate 2.7g	**1%**
Dietary Fiber 0.5g	**2%**
Total Sugars 1.8g	
Protein 0.3g	
Vitamin D 0mcg	0%
Calcium 7mg	1%
Iron 0mg	2%
Potassium 68mg	

Alfredo Sauce

PREP TIME: 10 minutes

COOK TIME: 10 minutes

SERVINGS: 8 (¼ cup per serving)

Ingredients:

- 2 tbsp butter (unsalted)
- ¼ tsp ground nutmeg
- 1 cup plain rice milk (rice milk)

- 1 ½ tbsp all purpose flour
- ¾ cup plain cream cheese
- 1 garlic clove (minced)
- 2 tbsp parmesan cheese
- ½ tsp ground black pepper

Directions:

1. Melt the butter in a sauce pan over medium heat.
2. Stir in the flour and minced garlic. Cook for about 2 minutes, stirring constantly.
3. Stir in the rice milk. Cook for about 4 minutes or until is thick, stirring constantly.
4. Add the cream cheese, nutmeg and parmesan cheese. Stir to combine and cook for 1 minute, stirring constantly until the sauce is smooth.
5. Remove the sauce pan from heat and stir in the ground black pepper.
6. Serve hot over kidney friendly pasta.

Nutrition Facts

Servings: 8

Amount per serving

Calories	**123**

% Daily Value*

Total Fat 9.8g	**13%**
Saturated Fat 6g	**30%**
Cholesterol 29mg	**10%**
Sodium 109mg	**5%**
Total Carbohydrate 7.6g	**3%**
Dietary Fiber 0.1g	**0%**
Total Sugars 2.9g	
Protein 3.1g	
Vitamin D 0mcg	1%
Calcium 100mg	8%
Iron 0mg	1%
Potassium 5mg	

Cinnamon Apple Sauce

PREP TIME: 10 minutes

COOK TIME: 30 minutes

SERVINGS: 6 servings (½ per serving)

Ingredients:

- 8 apples (peeled, cored and cut into chunks)
- 1/8 tsp ground all spice
- ½ cup water

148

- 1 tsp ground cinnamon
- ¼ tsp ground nutmeg
- ¼ tsp ground ginger

Directions:

1. Combine the apples, water, nutmeg, ginger, cinnamon and allspice in a large sauce pan over medium heat.
2. Cover the sauce pan and cook for about 15 to 20 minutes or until the apples are tender, stirring occasionally.
3. Remove the sauce from heat and use a potato mash to mash the apples.
4. Let the sauce cool completely before transferring it to jars for storage. Store in a refrigerator for up to 7 days.

Nutrition Facts

Servings: 6

Amount per serving

Calories	**12**

% Daily Value*

Total Fat 0.1g	0%
Saturated Fat 0g	0%
Cholesterol 0mg	0%
Sodium 1mg	0%
Total Carbohydrate 3.2g	1%
Dietary Fiber 0.5g	2%
Total Sugars 2.2g	
Protein 0.1g	
Vitamin D 0mcg	0%
Calcium 6mg	0%
Iron 0mg	0%
Potassium 23mg	

Italian Seasoning

PREP TIME: 5 minutes

SERVINGS: 24 (1/2 cup – 1 tsp per serving)

Ingredients:

- 2 tsp onion powder
- 1 tbsp oregano
- 2 tbsp garlic powder
- 1 tbsp parsley
- 1 tbsp basil

- 1/2tsp pepper
- ½ tsp thyme

Directions:

1. Combine all the ingredients in a small mixing bowl. Stir thoroughly until the ingredients are well combined.
2. Store in an airtight container.

Nutrition Facts

Servings: 24

Amount per serving

Calories	**4**

% Daily Value*

Total Fat 0g	**0%**
Saturated Fat 0g	**0%**
Cholesterol 0mg	**0%**
Sodium 0mg	**0%**
Total Carbohydrate 0.8g	**0%**
Dietary Fiber 0.2g	**1%**
Total Sugars 0.3g	
Protein 0.2g	
Vitamin D 0mcg	0%
Calcium 5mg	0%
Iron 0mg	1%
Potassium 15mg	

Breakfast

Blueberry Pancake

PREP TIME: 10 minutes

COOK TIME: 24 minutes

SERVINGS: 12 pancakes

Ingredients:

- 2 tbsp canola oil
- 2 eggs (beaten)
- 1 1/2cups sifted plain all purpose flour
- 1 cup buttermilk
- 1 tsp ground cinnamon
- 1 cup frozen blueberries (rinsed)
- 2 tsp Ener-G baking powder (or any other renal friendly sodium free baking powder)
- 3 tbsp sugar

Directions:

1. Sift the cinnamon, all-purpose flour and sugar into a large mixing bowl. Mix until the ingredients are well combined.
2. Use a spoon to make a hole in the middle of the mixture. Pour in the egg and buttermilk and mix until the mixture forms a smooth batter.
3. Fold in the rinsed blueberries.
4. Heat up a large pan and add little oil. Pour ½ cup of the batter into the pan.
5. Cook for about 1 to 2 minutes. Flip the pancake and cook the other side for about 1 to 2 minute too.
6. Repeat step 4 and 5 until all the batter has been cooked.
7. Serve and enjoy.

Nutrition Facts

Servings: 12

Amount per serving

Calories	**164**

% Daily Value*

Total Fat 3.4g	**4%**
Saturated Fat 0.5g	**3%**
Cholesterol 28mg	**9%**
Sodium 35mg	**2%**
Total Carbohydrate 30.2g	**11%**
Dietary Fiber 0.8g	**3%**
Total Sugars 5.3g	
Protein 2.1g	
Vitamin D 3mcg	13%
Calcium 204mg	16%
Iron 0mg	3%
Potassium 51mg	

Vegetable Omelet

PREP TIME: 5 minutes

COOK TIME: 5 minutes

SERVINGS: 1

Ingredients:

- 1 tbsp canola oil
- 1 whole egg

154

- 2 egg whites
- 2 tbsp water
- 1/3 cup frozen mixed vegetables
- 4 tbsp sliced green pepper
- ½ cup diced onion

Garnish:
- 2 fresh parsley sprigs (chopped)

Directions:

1. Cut the mixed vegetables into pieces and put them in a microwave safe dish. Add little water and cover the dish.
2. Place the dish in the microwave and microwave on HIGH for 2 minutes.
3. Remove the dish from the vegetables from the microwave and set them aside in a bowl.
4. Heat up the oil in a small nonstick skillet.
5. Add the onion and green pepper. Saute for about 2 minutes, stirring often.
6. Beat the egg, egg whites and water in a mixing bowl.
7. Pour the egg mixture into the skillet and cook until the egg is set and firm.
8. Add the mixed steamed mix vegetables and fold the omelet.
9. Remove the pan from heat.
10. Serve the omelet into plate and garnish with chop parsley.

Nutrition Facts

Servings: 1

Amount per serving

Calories	**270**

% Daily Value*

Total Fat 18.7g	**24%**
Saturated Fat 2.4g	**12%**
Cholesterol 164mg	**55%**
Sodium 216mg	**9%**
Total Carbohydrate 12g	**4%**
Dietary Fiber 3.3g	**12%**
Total Sugars 5.1g	
Protein 14.6g	
Vitamin D 15mcg	77%
Calcium 56mg	4%
Iron 1mg	8%
Potassium 378mg	

Pumpkin Pancake

PREP TIME: 10 minutes

COOK TIME: 15 minutes

SERVINGS: 8

Ingredients:

- 3 tbsp canola oil
- 2 cups gluten free baking flour
- 1 large egg (beaten)
- 1 tsp pure vanilla extract
- 2 tbsp pure maple syrup
- 1 tbsp Ener-G baking powder
- ½ tsp Ener-G baking soda
- 2 tbsp ground flax seeds
- ½ cup pumpkin puree (unsweetened)
- 1 ½ cup unsweetened almond milk
- ¼ tsp salt
- 1 tsp cinnamon

Directions:

1. In a large mixing bowl, combine the flour, baking powder, flax seeds, baking powder, cinnamon, salt and baking soda.
2. In another large mixing bowl, whisk together the egg, milk, vanilla extract, pumpkin puree and maple syrup.
3. Gently pour the wet ingredients into the dry ingredient, mixing as you pour in the wet ingredient. Mix until well combined and smooth.
4. Heat up a large skillet over medium to high heat.
5. Lightly oil the pan.
6. Pour about 1/3 cup of the batter into the pan.
7. Cook for about 1 to 2 minutes and flip. Cook the other side for about 1 to 2 minutes too.
8. Transfer the pancake to a neat plate.
9. Repeat the cooking process until all the batter has been cooked into pancakes.
10. Serve warm and enjoy.

Nutrition Facts

Servings: 8

Amount per serving

Calories	173

% Daily Value*

Total Fat 7.1g		**9%**
Saturated Fat 0.7g		**4%**
Cholesterol 23mg		**8%**
Sodium 118mg		**5%**
Total Carbohydrate 24.2g		**9%**
Dietary Fiber 2g		**7%**
Total Sugars 3.7g		
Protein 2.3g		
Vitamin D 2mcg		12%
Calcium 525mg		40%
Iron 4mg		22%
Potassium 102mg		

Granola Breakfast Bowl

PREP TIME: 10 minutes

COOK TIME: 25 minutes

SERVINGS: 5

Ingredients:

- 2 cups rolled oat
- ½ cup natural honey

- ¼ cup bee pollen
- 1 tsp vanilla extract
- ½ tsp salt or to taste
- 1 cup unsweetened reduced coconut flakes
- 3 tbsp coconut sugar
- 1 tsp cinnamon
- ¼ cup melted coconut oil
- ½ cup pecans (roughly chopped)
- ½ cup almonds (roughly chopped)

Topping:
- Almond milk

Directions:

1. Preheat your oven to 175°C.
2. Line a baking sheet with parchment paper, set aside.
3. Toss the oat into a large mixing bowl and add the chopped pecans, chopped almond, coconut sugar, coconut flakes, salt and cinnamon. Mix until the ingredients are evenly combined.
4. In another mixing bowl, mix the melted coconut oil, honey and vanilla extract.
5. Now, pour the honey mixture into the oat mixture and stir thoroughly until the ingredients are well combined.
6. Place the mixture on the line baking sheet and spread evenly, leveling the surface of the granola.
7. Place the baking sheet in the oven and bake for 15 minutes.
8. Remove the baking sheet from the oven and toss the granola mixture.
9. Return the baking sheet to the oven and bake for another 10 minutes.
10. Sprinkle the bee pollen over the roasted granola mixture and mix.
11. Lay parchment paper over the roasted granola and gently press the granola to the bottom of the baking sheet.
12. Remove and discard the parchment paper.

13. Leave the granola to cool for a few minutes.
14. Serve into bowls, top with almond milk and enjoy.

Nutrition Facts

Servings: 5

Amount per serving

Calories	518

% Daily Value*

Total Fat 34.5g	**44%**
Saturated Fat 9.1g	**45%**
Cholesterol 0mg	**0%**
Sodium 327mg	**14%**
Total Carbohydrate 44.1g	**16%**
Dietary Fiber 8.7g	**31%**
Total Sugars 3.2g	
Protein 10.1g	
Vitamin D 0mcg	0%
Calcium 63mg	5%
Iron 2mg	13%
Potassium 282mg	

Simple Cumin Raisin Breakfast Quinoa

PREP TIME: 5 minutes

COOK TIME: 17 minutes

SERVINGS: 8

Ingredients:

- 2 cups quinoa
- ½ cup raisins

- 2 tbsp cumin
- 4 cups vegetable broth
- 1 tbsp olive oil
- 1/2 tsp ground black pepper
- 1 small yellow onion (diced)

Garnish:

- 2 tbsp freshly chopped cilantro

Directions:

1. Heat up a pot on high heat and add oil.
2. Add the onions and saute until tender and lightly browned. This will take about 2 minutes.
3. Stir in the cumin, salt and pepper.
4. Pour in the broth and add the quinoa and raisin. Bring to a boil; reduce the heat and simmer for 10 to 15 minutes more.
5. Serve into bowls and garnish with chopped fresh cilantro.

Nutrition Facts

Servings: 8

Amount per serving

Calories	**227**

% Daily Value*

Total Fat 5.4g	**7%**
Saturated Fat 0.8g	**4%**
Cholesterol 0mg	**0%**
Sodium 388mg	**17%**
Total Carbohydrate 36.5g	**13%**
Dietary Fiber 3.7g	**13%**
Total Sugars 6.1g	
Protein 9.1g	
Vitamin D 0mcg	0%
Calcium 46mg	4%
Iron 3mg	19%
Potassium 453mg	

Blueberry Breakfast Smoothie Bowl

PREP TIME: 5 minutes

SERVINGS: 1 bowl

Ingredients:

- 1 cup frozen blueberries
- ½ tsp ginger
- ½ medium apple (peeled and slices)

- 1 tbsp fiber cereal
- 2 tbsp whey protein powder
- 100 g fat free Greek yogurt
- 1/3 cup unsweetened almond milk
- 5 raspberries
- 2 strawberries (sliced)
- 2 tsp shredded coconut

Directions:

1. Put blueberries and apple in a blender and blend until just smooth.
2. Add the almond milk, fiber cereal, protein powder, ginger and Greek yoghurt. Blend until smooth.
3. Serve the smoothie into bowl and top with shredded coconut, raspberry and strawberry

Nutrition Facts

Servings: 1

Amount per serving

Calories	**347**

% Daily Value*

Total Fat 5.6g	**7%**
Saturated Fat 1.9g	**10%**
Cholesterol 57mg	**19%**
Sodium 171mg	**7%**
Total Carbohydrate 54g	**20%**
Dietary Fiber 12.6g	**45%**
Total Sugars 27.8g	
Protein 26.3g	

Vitamin D 0mcg	2%
Calcium 140mg	11%
Iron 5mg	27%
Potassium 583mg	

Blueberry Muffin

PREP TIME: 15 minutes

COOK TIME: 30 minutes

SERVINGS: 12 muffins

Ingredients:

- 1/8 tsp ground ginger
- ½ cup canola oil

- 1 cup granulated sugar
- 2 cups fresh blueberries
- 2 cups unsweetened rice milk
- 2 tbsp pure vanilla extract
- 1tbsp Ener-G baking soda (or any other renal friendly sodium free baking powder)
- ½ tsp ground nutmeg
- 1 tsp cinnamon
- 3 ½ cups all-purpose flour

Directions:

1. Preheat the oven to 375°F and line 12 muffin cups with parchment paper.
2. In a large mixing bowl, combine the all-purpose flour, nutmeg, cinnamon, baking powder, ginger and sugar. Mix until the ingredients are well combined.
3. In another large mixing bowl, combine the vanilla extract, rice milk and canola oil. Mix until well combined.
4. Now, pour the milk mixture into the flour mixture and mix until you form a smooth batter.
5. Fold in the blueberries.
6. Fill each muffin cup with the batter. The muffin cups should not be filled to the beam; leave at least 1 inch empty.
7. Arrange the muffin cups into a baking sheet and place the baking sheet into the oven.
8. Bake for about 25 minutes to 30 minutes or until a toothpick inserted in the middle of the muffin comes out clean.
9. Remove the muffins from the oven and leave them to cool.
10. Remove the muffins from the muffin cups and serve.
11. Enjoy.

Nutrition Facts

Servings: 12

Amount per serving

Calories	**317**

% Daily Value*

Total Fat 10g	**13%**
Saturated Fat 0.8g	**4%**
Cholesterol 0mg	**0%**
Sodium 18mg	**1%**
Total Carbohydrate 52.3g	**19%**
Dietary Fiber 1.7g	**6%**
Total Sugars 21.1g	
Protein 4.1g	
Vitamin D 0mcg	1%
Calcium 71mg	5%
Iron 2mg	12%
Potassium 66mg	

Overnight French toast

PREP TIME: 20 minutes

COOK TIME: 50 minutes

SERVINGS: 9

Ingredients:

- 1 loaf of white bread (cut into 1 inch slices)
- ½ cup unsweetened dried blueberries

- 1 tbsp vanilla
- 3 tsp cinnamon
- 1 tsp nutmeg
- 3 apples (peeled, cored, and finely chopped)
- 1 ½ cups unsweetened rice milk
- 6 eggs
- ½ cup margarine (unsalted)
- 1 cup brown sugar

Directions:

1. Whisk together the brown sugar, 1 tsp cinnamon, nutmeg and mayonnaise in a 13 by 9 inch dish.
2. Add the blueberries and apple. Toss until well combined.
3. Toss until the ingredients are well combined.
4. Spread the mixture and press it to the bottom of the baking dish.
5. Arrange with bread slices on the apple mixture.
6. In a large mixing bowl, whisk together the eggs, rice milk, 2 tsp cinnamon and vanilla.
7. Pour the egg mixture over the bread slices in the baking dish. Cover the baking dish with foil and place it in a refrigerator. Refrigerate the mixture overnight.
8. Preheat the oven to 375°F.
9. Place the baking dish in the oven and bake for about 40 minutes, covered.
10. Remove the baking dish from the oven and uncover the dish.
11. Return the dish to the oven and bake the toast for another 5 minutes.
12. After the baking cycle, remove the baking dish from the oven and let the toast cool for about 5 minutes.
13. Serve the French toast and enjoy.

Nutrition Facts

Servings: 9

Amount per serving

Calories	**588**

% Daily Value*

Total Fat 26.1g	**33%**
Saturated Fat 4.5g	**23%**
Cholesterol 109mg	**36%**
Sodium 500mg	**22%**
Total Carbohydrate 75.9g	**28%**
Dietary Fiber 3.6g	**13%**
Total Sugars 32.1g	
Protein 11.6g	
Vitamin D 10mcg	52%
Calcium 224mg	17%
Iron 4mg	20%
Potassium 174mg	

Cinnamon Bran Muffins

PREP TIME: 10 minutes

COOK TIME: 20 minutes

SERVINGS: 12

Ingredients:

- 1 tsp cinnamon
- 1 egg

- 1 tsp pure vanilla extract
- 1 ½ tsp Ener-G sodium free baking soda (or any other kidney friendly sodium free baking soda)
- 1/3 cup natural honey
- 1 cup wheat bran
- ¼ tsp cream of tartar
- 1 cup crushed pineapple (drained)
- 1cup all-purpose flour

Directions:

1. Preheat the oven to 400°F and grease 12 muffin cups.
2. In a large mixing bowl, combine the cinnamon, all-purpose flour, wheat bran, cream of tartar and baking soda.
3. In another large mixing, combine the crushed pineapple, honey, egg and vanilla extract.
4. Now, pour the flour mixture into the egg mixture and mix until you form a smooth barter.
5. Fill each muffin cup with the batter. The muffin cups should not be filled to the beam; leave at least 1 inch empty.
6. Arrange the muffin cups into a baking sheet and place the baking sheet into the oven.
7. Bake for about 25 minutes to 30 minutes or until a toothpick inserted in the middle of the muffin comes out clean.
8. Remove the muffins from the oven and leave them to cool.
9. Remove the muffins from the muffin cups and serve.
10. Enjoy.

Nutrition Facts

Servings: 12

Amount per serving

Calories	**63**

% Daily Value*

Total Fat 0.6g	**1%**
Saturated Fat 0.1g	**1%**
Cholesterol 14mg	**5%**
Sodium 5mg	**0%**
Total Carbohydrate 13.3g	**5%**
Dietary Fiber 2.7g	**10%**
Total Sugars 2.2g	
Protein 2.3g	
Vitamin D 1mcg	6%
Calcium 16mg	1%
Iron 1mg	6%
Potassium 88mg	

Corn Pudding

PREP TIME: 10 minutes

COOK TIME: 40 minutes

SERVINGS: 6

Ingredients:

- 2 tbsp granulated sugar
- 3 eggs (beaten)

- 2 tbsp all-purpose flour
- ½ tsp Ener-G baking soda (or any other renal friendly sodium free baking soda)
- ¾ cup rice milk (unsweetened)
- 2 cups frozen corn kernels (defrosted)
- 2 tbsp sour cream
- 1 tsp pure vanilla extract
- 3 tbsp unsalted butter (softened)
- 1 tsp ginger powder

Directions:

1. Preheat your oven to 350°F and grease and 8 by 8 inch baking dish with butter.
2. In a large mixing bowl, combine the egg, rice milk, sugar, butter, sour cream and vanilla extract. Mix until the ingredients are well combined.
3. In another mixing bowl, combine the all-purpose flour, ginger baking soda.
4. Pour the flour mixture into the egg mixture and mix until you form a smooth batter.
5. Add the defrosted corn and mix until well combined.
6. Fill the prepared baking dish with the batter.
7. Place the baking dish in the preheated oven and bake for about 40 minutes.
8. After the baking cycle, remove the baking dish from the oven and let the pudding cool for about 12 to 15 minutes.
9. Serve the corn pudding into bowls and enjoy.

Nutrition Facts

Servings: 6

Amount per serving

Calories	**177**

% Daily Value*

Total Fat 9.5g	**12%**
Saturated Fat 4.9g	**25%**
Cholesterol 99mg	**33%**
Sodium 87mg	**4%**
Total Carbohydrate 19.9g	**7%**
Dietary Fiber 1.4g	**5%**
Total Sugars 7.3g	
Protein 4.8g	
Vitamin D 12mcg	59%
Calcium 62mg	5%
Iron 1mg	5%
Potassium 175mg	

Breakfast Meatballs

PREP TIME: 20 minutes

COOK TIME: 25 minutes

SERVINGS: 35 meatballs

Ingredients:

- 1pound lean ground turkey
- ¼ cup finely chopped onions
- 1tsp hot sauce

- ½ tsp garlic powder
- 1tsp sodium free poultry seasoning
- ¼ tsp dry mustard
- 1 tsp granulated sugar
- 1/2 tsp onion powder
- 1 tbsp fresh lemon juice
- 1 tsp Italian seasoning

Sauce ingredients:
- 2 cups of water
- ¼ cup vegetable oil
- 1tsp curry
- 1 tsp hot sauce
- 2 tbsp all-purpose flour
- 2 tsp vinegar
- 1 tsp onion powder

Garnish:
- Chopped fresh parsley (optional)

Directions:

1. Preheat your oven to 425°F and line a baking sheet with parchment paper.
2. In a large mixing bowl, combine the ground turkey, chopped onions, sugar lemon juice.
3. Add the Italian seasoning, onion powder, hot sauce, mustard, garlic powder and poultry seasoning. Mix until well combined.
4. Use a tablespoon to scoop out equal amount of the mixture and mold into balls.
5. Arrange the meatballs into the lined baking sheet in a single layer.
6. Place the baking sheet in the preheated oven and bake the meatballs for about 20 minutes or until the meatballs are done.

7. Meanwhile, prepare the sauce. Place a sauce pan on heat and add the vegetable oil and all-purpose flour.
8. Cook for a few minutes, stirring constantly until the mixture is slightly browned.
9. Remove the saucepan from heat and stir in the onion powder, hot sauce, water, curry and sugar.
10. Return the saucepan to heat and cook until the sauce thickens, stirring constantly. Remove the saucepan from heat.
11. After the baking cycle, remove the baking sheet from the oven and leave the meatballs to cool for a few minutes.
12. Serve the meatballs warm with the sauce and garnish with chopped fresh parsley.

Nutrition Facts

Servings: 35

Amount per serving

Calories	**36**

% Daily Value*

Total Fat 2.6g	**3%**
Saturated Fat 0.4g	**2%**
Cholesterol 9mg	**3%**
Sodium 18mg	**1%**
Total Carbohydrate 0.7g	**0%**
Dietary Fiber 0.1g	**0%**
Total Sugars 0.2g	
Protein 2.6g	
Vitamin D 0mcg	0%
Calcium 4mg	0%
Iron 0mg	1%
Potassium 48mg	1%

Breakfast Frittata

PREP TIME: 15 minutes

COOK TIME: 35 minutes

SERVINGS: 6

Ingredients:

- 8 eggs
- 1 tbsp vegetable oil

- 1 cup chopped asparagus
- 1/8 tsp garlic
- ¼ tsp onion powder
- 1/4 tsp salt
- ½ tsp ground black pepper
- 1/8 tsp cayenne pepper
- 1/8 tsp cumin
- 1/8 tsp coriander
- 1/8 tsp oregano
- 1 red bell pepper (seeded and chopped)
- ½ tsp dried basil
- ½ cup shredded Swiss cheese
- ½ cup rice milk
- 1 medium potato (peeled and cut into bite sizes) *See notes

Directions:

1. Put the potato pieces in a pot and add enough water.
2. Bring the water and potato to a boil.
3. Drain off the hot water and add fresh water.
4. Bring the fresh water and potatoes to a boil and cook until the potato pieces are tender.
5. Drain the water and set aside.
6. In a mixing bowl, whisk together the egg, basil, rice milk, oregano, coriander, cayenne pepper, black pepper, salt, onion powder and garlic. Set aside.
7. Heat up the vegetable oil in a frying pan over medium to high heat.
8. Add the chopped pepper and asparagus and saute until the vegetables are tender, stirring often.
9. Add the cooked potato pieces and stir. Spread out the veggies and potato across the pan.
10. Pour the egg mixture over the ingredients in the frying pan.
11. Cover the pan, reduce the heat and cook for about 15 minutes or until the eggs are set and the frittata is firm.

12. Sprinkle the Swiss cheese over the frittata after the first 13 minutes of cooking.
13. Remove the frying pan from heat and let the frittata cool for a few minutes.
14. Cut frittata into sizes and serve.

Note: it is important that you double cook the potatoes as instructed. Changing the water after the first boiling helps to reduce the potatoes' potassium content. Preparing this recipe without double boiling the potatoes will turn the meal into a high potassium meal.

Nutrition Facts

Servings: 6

Amount per serving

Calories	**188**

% Daily Value*

Total Fat 10.9g	**14%**
Saturated Fat 3.9g	**20%**
Cholesterol 227mg	**76%**
Sodium 207mg	**9%**
Total Carbohydrate 11.9g	**4%**
Dietary Fiber 1.6g	**6%**
Total Sugars 2.3g	
Protein 11.3g	
Vitamin D 24mcg	122%
Calcium 118mg	9%
Iron 2mg	11%
Potassium 329mg	

Egg Sandwiches

PREP TIME: 5 minutes

COOK TIME: 20 minutes

SERVINGS: 6 sandwiches

Ingredients:

- 8 small eggs
- 12 slices of bread

- 2 green onions (chopped)
- ½ cup finely chopped celery
- 1/3 cup light sour cream
- 1 tbsp mayonnaise
- ¼ cup chopped green pepper
- 1/8 tsp paprika
- 1/8 tsp ground black pepper
- ¼ tsp ground mustard

Directions:

1. Place the eggs in a pot and add enough water.
2. Bring the egg and to a rolling boil over high heat, reduce the heat and cook for 15 minutes to ensure the eggs are hard boiled.
3. Remove eggs from heat and put them in a bowl of cold water for a few minutes. Peel the eggs.
4. Place the peeled eggs in a bowl and mash.
5. Now, add the mayonnaise, sour cream, paprika, green pepper, onion, celery and mustard. Mix until the ingredients are well combined.
6. Arrange six bread slices on a tray and spoon equal amount of the egg mixture onto the bread.
7. Spread the egg mixture and cover the bread slices with the remaining bread slices.
8. Serve and enjoy.

Nutrition Facts

Servings: 6

Amount per serving

Calories	**162**

% Daily Value*

Total Fat 9g	**12%**
Saturated Fat 3.5g	**18%**
Cholesterol 195mg	**65%**
Sodium 226mg	**10%**
Total Carbohydrate 11.5g	**4%**
Dietary Fiber 0.8g	**3%**
Total Sugars 1.9g	
Protein 8.4g	
Vitamin D 42mcg	208%
Calcium 79mg	6%
Iron 2mg	9%
Potassium 151mg	

Carrot Scramble

PREP TIME: 10 minutes

COOK TIME: 10 minutes

SERVINGS: 4

Ingredients:

- 2 tbsp olive oil
- 5 eggs (beaten)

- 1/4tsp garlic powder
- 1/8 tsp basil
- 1/8 tsp pepper
- 1 cup chopped onion
- ½ cup nestle non dairy creamer
- 1 cup cooked carrot
- ½ medium red pepper (chopped)
- ¼ cup frozen corn (defrosted)

Directions:

1. Heat up the olive oil in a skillet over medium to high heat.
2. Add the onion and chopped pepper. Saute until the onion is browned and tender, stirring often.
3. Add the carrot, corn, pepper, garlic powder and basil. Stir and cook for about 2 minutes.
4. In a mixing bowl, whisk together the eggs and non dairy creamer.
5. Pour the egg mixture into the pan and cook until the eggs are set.
6. Remove the skillet from heat and serve the scramble.
7. Enjoy.

Nutrition Facts

Servings: 4

Amount per serving

Calories	**214**

% Daily Value*

Total Fat 14.6g	**19%**
Saturated Fat 2.7g	**14%**
Cholesterol 205mg	**68%**
Sodium 99mg	**4%**
Total Carbohydrate 12.8g	**5%**
Dietary Fiber 1.8g	**6%**
Total Sugars 6g	
Protein 8g	
Vitamin D 19mcg	96%
Calcium 47mg	4%
Iron 1mg	8%
Potassium 261mg	

Eggplant Casserole

PREP TIME: 15 minutes

COOK TIME: 55 minutes

SERVINGS: 8

Ingredients:

- 1 large egg (lightly beaten)
- 1tsp Italian seasoning

- 1 clove garlic (crushed)
- 1 large eggplant (peeled)
- 2 cups plain bread crumbs
- 1 pound lean ground turkey
- 2 tbsp olive oil
- ½ tsp red pepper
- ½ cup green pepper (chopped)
- ½ cup finely chopped onion

Directions:

1. Preheat the oven to 350°F.
2. Place the peeled eggplant in a pot and add enough water.
3. Bring the eggplant and water to a rolling boil and cook until the eggplant is tender.
4. Put the eggplant in a bowl and mash it.
5. Heat up the olive oil in a large skillet over medium to high heat.
6. Add the garlic, onion, green pepper and ground turkey. Saute until the ground turkey is cooked.
7. Add the egg, mashed eggplant and breadcrumbs.
8. Add Italian seasoning and red pepper. Mix until the ingredients are well combined.
9. Pour the mixture in the skillet into a casserole dish.
10. Place the casserole dish in the preheated oven and bake for about 40 to 45 minutes.
11. After the baking cycle, remove the casserole from the oven and let it cool for a few minutes.
12. Serve warm and enjoy

Nutrition Facts

Servings: 8

Amount per serving

Calories	**253**

% Daily Value*

Total Fat 10g	**13%**
Saturated Fat 2.5g	**13%**
Cholesterol 64mg	**21%**
Sodium 254mg	**11%**
Total Carbohydrate 25.1g	**9%**
Dietary Fiber 3.4g	**12%**
Total Sugars 4.7g	
Protein 16.7g	
Vitamin D 2mcg	11%
Calcium 62mg	5%
Iron 2mg	13%
Potassium 363mg	

Meatloaf (no sauce)

PREP TIME: 15 minutes

COOK TIME: 45 minutes

SERVINGS: 8

Ingredients:

- ½ cup water
- ¼ cup carrots (cooked, drained and finely chopped)

- 2 celery stalks (finely chopped)
- ¼ tsp black pepper
- 1/2tsp onion powder
- ½ cup plain breadcrumbs
- 1 tbsp fresh lemon juice
- ½ tsp Italian seasoning
- ¼ tsp oregano
- Half green pepper (diced)
- 1 small onion (diced)

Directions:

1. Preheat the oven to 400°F and grease loaf pan.
2. Put the ground turkey in a mixing bowl and add the lemon juice. Mix until well combined.
3. Add the diced onion, green pepper, onion powder, black pepper, bread crumbs, carrot, celery and Italian seasoning.
4. Pour water the ingredients in the mixing bowl and mix until the ingredients are well combined.
5. Mold the mixture into a meatloaf and place it in the loaf pan.
6. Place the loaf pan in the preheated oven and bake for about 45 minutes.
7. After the baking cycle, remove the loaf pan and let the meatloaf sit for a few minutes to cool.
8. Cut into slices and serve.

Nutrition Facts

Servings: 8

Amount per serving

Calories	36

% Daily Value*

Total Fat 0.5g	**1%**
Saturated Fat 0.1g	**1%**

Cholesterol 0mg	**0%**
Sodium 57mg	**2%**
Total Carbohydrate 6.8g	**2%**
Dietary Fiber 0.8g	**3%**
Total Sugars 1.3g	
Protein 1.2g	
Vitamin D 0mcg	0%
Calcium 20mg	2%
Iron 0mg	2%
Potassium 67mg	

Renal friendly lunch, dinner and soups

Creamy Celery Soup

PREP TIME: 10 minutes

COOK TIME: 20 minutes

SERVINGS: 8

Ingredients:

- 1 tbsp olive oil
- 4 cups chopped celery
- 2 cups chopped yellow onion
- 1 tsp Italian seasoning
- 1 tbsp freshly chopped thyme
- ¼ tsp salt

- 1 tbsp fresh lemon juice
- 1/2 cup heavy cream
- 1/8 tsp ground black pepper
- 4 cups unsalted chicken broth
- 1 tsp lemon zest
- 1 tsp cumin
- 2 cups fresh baby spinach
- 4 garlic cloves (crushed)

Garnish:
- 2 tbsp fresh chopped parsley

Directions:

1. Heat up 1 tbsp olive oil in a large pot over medium to high heat.
2. Add the onions, celery, thyme and garlic.
3. Saute for about 10 minutes or until the vegetables are soft, stirring constantly.
4. Stir in the lemon zest, cumin and Italian seasoning.
5. Pour in the chicken broth and add salt.
6. Bring the soup to a boil, reduce the heat and simmer for 6 minutes or until the celery pieces are tender.
7. Add the lemon juice and spinach. Cook for 2 minutes.
8. Remove the pot from heat and use a hand blender to puree the soup until smooth.
9. If you do not have a hand blender, let the soup cool for a few minutes, transfer it to a regular blender and blend until smooth. After blending return the soup to the pot.
10. Stir in the heavy whipping cream and black pepper.
11. Serve soup into bowls and garnish with chopped fresh parsley.
12. Enjoy.

Nutrition Facts

Servings: 8

Amount per serving

Calories	**61**

% Daily Value*

Total Fat 5g	**6%**
Saturated Fat 2.1g	**10%**
Cholesterol 11mg	**4%**
Sodium 125mg	**5%**
Total Carbohydrate 3.7g	**1%**
Dietary Fiber 1.4g	**5%**
Total Sugars 1.2g	
Protein 1g	
Vitamin D 4mcg	20%
Calcium 48mg	4%
Iron 1mg	6%
Potassium 212mg	

Cucumber Shrimp Soup

PREP TIME: 20 minutes

SERVINGS: 4

Ingredients:

- 1 cup shallot
- ¼ tsp crushed red pepper
- 2 medium cucumber (peeled, seeded and chopped)

- ¼ cup radishes (finely chopped)
- 4 tbsp chopped fresh parsley
- 2 whole garlic cloves (crushed)
- 2 cups unsweetened almond milk
- 3 tbsp fresh lemon juice
- ¼ lemon pepper seasoning
- 8 ounces shrimp (peeled, deveined, cooked and chopped)
- 2 tbsp red wine vinegar
- 1 cup plain fat free Greek yogurt

Directions:

1. Toss the cucumber into a powerful blender and add almond milk, Greek yogurt, lemon juice, crushed red pepper, lemon pepper seasoning, garlic, shallot and parsley. Blend until smooth.
2. Now, the blended mixture into a large mixing bowl.
3. Add the chopped shrimp, vinegar and radishes. Mix until well combined.
4. Place the mixing bowl in a refrigerator and chill the soup for a few minutes.
5. Serve soup into bowls and enjoy.

Nutrition Facts

Servings: 4

Amount per serving

Calories	**173**

% Daily Value*

Total Fat 3.2g	**4%**
Saturated Fat 0.6g	**3%**
Cholesterol 121mg	**40%**
Sodium 272mg	**12%**
Total Carbohydrate 14.6g	**5%**
Dietary Fiber 1.6g	**6%**
Total Sugars 4.1g	
Protein 21.4g	
Vitamin D 1mcg	3%
Calcium 417mg	32%
Iron 2mg	9%
Potassium 527mg	

Ground beef Soup

PREP TIME: 35 minutes

COOK TIME: 10 minutes

SERVINGS: 6

Ingredients:

- ½ cup onion
- 1tsp allspice

- 1 tbsp fresh lemon juice
- ½ tsp ground black pepper
- 1/3 cup white rice (uncooked)
- 1 tsp hot sauce
- 2 cups water
- 3 cups frozen mixed vegetables (unsalted)
- 1 tbsp sour cream
- 1 cup low sodium beef broth

Directions:

1. Heat up a large saucepan over medium to high heat.
2. Add the onion ground beef and saute until the ground beef and onion are browned, stirring often. Drain the beef fat.
3. Pour in the water and add the allspice, lemon juice, pepper, hot sauce, mixed vegetables, broth and rice.
4. Bring the soup to a boil, cover the saucepan, reduce the heat and simmer the soup for30 minutes.
5. Remove the saucepan from heat and stir in the sour cream.
6. Serve and enjoy.

Nutrition Facts

Servings: 6

Amount per serving

Calories	**113**

% Daily Value*

Total Fat 0.9g	**1%**
Saturated Fat 0.4g	**2%**
Cholesterol 1mg	**0%**
Sodium 185mg	**8%**
Total Carbohydrate 21.7g	**8%**
Dietary Fiber 4.5g	**16%**
Total Sugars 3.4g	
Protein 4.4g	
Vitamin D 0mcg	0%
Calcium 37mg	3%
Iron 1mg	8%
Potassium 228mg	